LIVING BEYOND OUR SELL BY DATE

…and growing older disgracefully!

LIVING BEYOND OUR SELL BY DATE

…and growing older disgracefully!

Living Beyond Our Sell by Date is the book of "someday" for those of us who are growing older disgracefully.

Evelyn Marder Levin, PhD

Copyright © 2015 by Evelyn Marder Levin, PhD

All rights reserved. This book or any portion thereof may not be reproduced or used in any manner whatsoever without the express written permission of the author except for the use of brief quotations in a book review.

Printed in the United States of America

First Printing, 2015

ISBN-10:   1-506-13380-0

ISBN-13:   978-1-50613-380-5

www.grrouch.com
evelyn@grrouch.com

Printed by CreateSpace

Acknowledgements

A special thanks to those who helped me in many different ways: Betty Bishop, Justin Harter, Rosemary Vanderwyde, Paula Walker, and Kim Whetstone

… and for those who left too soon: Karen Ness, Keith Relkin

CONTENTS

1. Our Sell by Date 1
2. Grouch 5
3. Time to Retire or to Retread? 10
4. We Have Seen the Glory 13
5. Let's Hear It for Generation Speak 16
6. Where Have All the People Gone? 18
7. A Son Is a Son 21
8. You Don't Bring Me Flowers 24
9. What's up Doc? 27
10. Who Fixes Your Income? 30
11. Just a Simple Fish Story 33
12. Advice with Consent 36
13. Time on Our Hands 39
14. A Vote Is a Terrible Thing to Waste 43
15. Kicking the Habit 45
16. Kermit, Kermit, Where Is My Permit? 48
17. Let's Hear It like It Is 51
18. Kind: A Forgotten Four Letter Word? 54
19. The Pecking Order 57
20. Mother's Day -- A Commercial Holiday? 61
21. If Only 64
22. The Informers 67

23. Hurry up and Slow Down..70
24. Shoot the Messenger, Please! 73
25. When Is Enough, Enough?..77
26. Bone Loss, Not Retirement, Diminishes 80
27. Where's the Equality?...84
28. Grow Old along with Me, the Rest Is yet to Be 87
29. The Eye of the Beholder 90
30. Too Late Smart?...93
31. Why Is It so Hard to Be Kind? 96
32. Whee! Are Family..99
33. They Have Their Hands in Your Pockets 102
34. Silk Purse or Sow's Ear?..105
35. Love in the Afternoon 107
36. Welcome to Happy Hour..110
37. Day Life Savings Time 113
38. The Body Has a Head 116
39. Valentine's Day – What's Love Got to Do with It?....119
40. If You Were the Only Boy 122
41. Stand Your Ground……..Oh, Do Sit Down 125
42. Dream, When You're Feeling Blue 128
43. Boots Are made for Walking..130
44. The Wizard of Oz..133
45. To Resolve or Not to Resolve 136

46. I Know How You Feel …. Do Youooooo? 139

47. Delayed Gratification 141

48. Happy Holiday, All Right, Already 144

49. It's Airport Scan, Not Scam 147

50. Reach out and Touch Someone 150

51. Animal Crackers in My Soup 153

52. Opposable Thumbs, Who Needs Them? 156

53. Putting on the Dog 159

54. All in the Family 162

55. Elephants: Aging with Grace 165

56. Only the Lonely 168

57. My Car Comes Clean 171

58. Where Did My Little Wheels Go? 174

59. Recipe for Living 177

60. IS Thicker Than 180

61. What Price Dignity? Respect? 183

62. Happiness 185

1. OUR SELL BY DATE

Once upon a time, living to a great age was just about every one's goal in life. And what was a great age, anyway? Well, 60, 70 or even 80, if you were so blessed with the right genes or whatever else it took to remain on earth beyond your sell by date.

Your sell by date?

Now really, are we a carton of milk or a container of juice (in case we're lactose intolerant)? Very funny, but somewhat insulting, I have to say. Human beings have no expiration date as such, but for decades, actuarial tables, based on longevity statistics, have allowed most of the world to predict how much will have to be spent on aging human beings or to be more accurate, on human beings as they get older and older and older. In the senior complex where I live, a friend's mother celebrated her 100th birthday last year. My friend contacted the local newspaper, hoping they would come out to interview her mother

"But what does she do?" the reporter asked.

Surprised by the question, my friend answered, "She walks, talks, reads - what everyone does."

"That's the problem", the reporter replied. "We have so many octogenarians these days, that unless they do something special, we can't interview them all."

In 1929, life expectancy at birth - for women - was 60 years of age. Today, our life expectancy is 77.77 years of age. I've chosen the ladies because they live longer and because I admit to a certain bias as a member of the clan. So when legislation was passed by a government, in a well-meaning gesture of benevolence to its citizenry, there were mixed feelings, as always, but as time elapsed, on balance, the gesture grew from its position of acceptance to, it's okay for now, but can't you get us more money?

The legislation to which I refer, was the Social Security Act of 1935 and the timing of the Act was perfect, because it came on the heels of the great depression which had left millions impoverished and unemployed. The President, at that time, was Franklin

D. Roosevelt, and interestingly, though himself from an exceedingly wealthy and privileged background, he was concerned with protection for the unemployed, the poor and the elderly. Actually, that's not so surprising. When you are poor yourself, your energy is usually focused on trying to be "unpoor" and your charitable side is turned inward.

I digress. In Roosevelt's State of the Union Address, he said, "we have not weeded out the over privileged and we have not effectively lifted up the underprivileged."

One of the basic reasons the Act came into being, was for the protection of the disabled as well as the elderly, from the expenses of illnesses for which it would be impossible for them to pay, without totally depleting any savings they might have put aside, assuming they even had savings. The original Social Security Act involved numerous Titles, and six of the Titles pertained to programs including old age assistance, old age retirement benefits, unemployment compensation, aid to dependent children, and aid to the blind. Remaining programs included the Social Security Board; methods of taxation to pay for the program, and as usual, there were the issues of Federal versus state and local control.

We're living longer and retiring younger, and we're caught in the squeeze of too little money and too much time. For too little money, there are government agencies and philanthropic charities and a general awareness that a problem exists. We all understand how not having sufficient money to meet our needs, impacts our lives. However, an excess of time seems like a blessing to people who have spent most of their lives in a time warp, in which there is never enough time and whose mantra has been, some day when I have time.

Living Beyond Our Sell By Date is the book of "someday" for those of us who are growing older disgracefully. Living beyond our sell by date has to be lived, to be experienced. It cannot be imagined, and so in the pages that follow, are words from someone who is experiencing the time of now.

2. GROUCH

Who am I, anyway?

Call me a grouch. You probably think I am. The reason? I have decided to grow older disgracefully and that means breaking lots of rules - some of yours - some of mine.

I've probably arrived at the time of Social Security and maybe Medicare. I'm not a prophet of doom, but actuarially, if you have lived sixty years, you probably won't live another sixty. Those promises you have been making to yourself about future actions, will have less chance for actual fulfillment, so stop the damned procrastination. Do it now. Forget about quantity and start focusing on the quality of your life. All stuff that we'll talk about more as we go on, and we grouches do go on.

Forget about the mañana syndrome. You know

how that goes. I will do it tomorrow or at least someday, maybe the same someday when that prince or princess comes along. Forget all those terrible rules enslaving you as to what to do, and when and how to do it. Like so many of us, you wanted to fit in with the group to which you had attached yourself. Fitting in meant doing the same thing as ninety-eight percent of what the rest of your world was doing. Your self-confidence came partly from that feeling of belonging, and the belief that you could rectify past mistakes with future actions. Forget it. You have reached the promised land and in the words of the playwright, Robert Burton, "No rule is so general which admits not to some exception." Just a fancy way to say that rules are made to be broken and I might add, what better time than now?

Yes, fellow grouches, this is the time to be outspoken, to make up for all the years when you were mute for some reason or other. As a grandparent, we can be outspoken when we see some child's ego being trampled on by an irate or impatient parent, and ream out the so-called grown up instead. If our adult children are embarrassed by our behavior, it's obviously our fault for not bringing them up right, and they can always resort to mutterings of dementia, along with pitying looks in our direction. We don't care. We know where the true dementia lies.

We don't have to suck it up when some clerk in a store is rude, surly, or with an attitude that's as big as all outdoors. It's too late to teach them what they should have learned in pre-school, but it's okay to show them that you're not pleased. Sometimes, I'll ask if they're having a bad day. If they inquire as to why I'm asking, I'll say that they seem mad or sad or whatever. Some interesting replies and reactions to that. If I'm feeling really bitchy, I ask for their name and the name of their manager and mutter unintelligibly. If I'm with a friend, I just talk about them as if they were invisible and invisible people can't speak, all they do is just fume.

I use the age card a lot a lot a lot. It took a long time to get to this place and though I can still hear and see pretty well, I find it hard to deal with someone who thinks that anyone over forty is senile and anyone over sixty can't possibly be still breathing. Stating your age and looking apologetically at your interrogator works most places, except when the entire population is elderly. What you say and how you say it doesn't matter as much as just saying it. Age may have diminished our stature - so many of us are defined by our disintegrating bones - but it doesn't mean that we are any less agile with our minds.

Absolutely, and that's where we grouches step

up. For what seems like forever, we have had it drilled into our heads that seniors, especially women, should age gracefully. What exactly does that mean? Keeping our mouths shut no matter what? Taking whatever is handed to us? Accepting second rate services because we are getting older and therefore, less important in the scheme of things? No, no, no and no!

We have the maturity and wisdom to break the rules and we should. Don't get me wrong. I'm not advocating that you all become lawbreakers. It's hard enough to get a night's sleep on our firm inner springs, let alone deal with a mattress in a cell. What I'm referring to are society's often meaningless rules, predicated on some lines in our faces and gray in our hair.

Many of us have raised families and devoted our lives to others, but this should be our time, the time we think about ourselves without feelings of guilt. Of course we know about those feelings and we know lots more. We're going to think about letting our hair grow down to our butts, if it pleases us, and slathering on tons of eye makeup, if it makes us happy, and wearing short skirts if we feel good about our legs - or not. – In short, we're going to make our own rules and we'll have some old fogies like ourselves – give us their advice and their stories. I hope you'll all become a part of us with your own opinions and experiences. We're going to have fun and make these the best years of our lives. Think about it. Growing older disgracefully. You can't get a better mantra than that.

And now, to the words that pertain to those of us who are living beyond our sell by date.

3. TIME TO RETIRE OR TO RETREAD?

It used to be - across the board - when you reached a certain age - you retired. Ah yes, you had reached the promised land and for the rest of your life you could do nothing, or something of your own choosing. In your mind, the years stretched ahead like holiday lights on a string and you were in a celebratory mood. But then, the lights began to dim and the string stretched out more and more and what happened to that party, anyway?

I'll tell you what. Time, like any good thing, became too much and you couldn't use it all up. You know, leftovers are good the next day or so, but after that, you have to seriously think about pitching them. Easier said than done as I, and many of us who have been growing older disgracefully, have found out.

On the other hand, if you took early retirement, so to speak, and planned to find a second career for yourself, you might just be ahead of the game. For example, if you spent your life behind a desk crunching numbers, and were feeling down for the count, this might be your moment or many moments, in fact, to do something entirely different. Of course your physical condition might impact your choice, but setting that aside, maybe this is the moment to consider life as a ski instructor or maybe, after watching the Academy Awards, you realize that it's not too late for a few acting lessons, leading to a career trodding the boards, as we say.

The point is- and there is a point, as always, to my rambles - retiring too early is not a fast track to the yellow brick road which, when your feet are traversing it, stretches on and on and on. Get my drift? You need a destination. The part of your life, which is behind you, was probably filled with all sorts of things and you had a focus - places to go, people to see. You moaned and groaned, but you were never at loose ends, finding ways to kill the time, which you never seemed to have.

We are growing older, but in our heads we are the young old, and we may fill a rocking chair once in a while, but our minds haven't gone to sleep. So, we must find ways to occupy ourselves. To keep on working, if we're able and willing, is one cause for gratitude. To retire at will and not when society wills it, is another. Retirement should have meaning and every day should be part of that string of holiday lights. Really, what 's more glorious than the words, I've got the world on a string? My world? Or your world? Or just the whole darn world?

4. WE HAVE SEEN THE GLORY

It's one of those days, just one of those days. You know, the kind where doing anything is almost more than you can bear. Tomorrow I'll do it, you told yourself the day before, forgetting how fast tomorrows come, and it's here now and you can bite the bullet. Or not. But you've always been a biter, so you hit the glory road.

Only now you see it, now you don't. My eyes begin their fight with my computer. Am I too enlightened? So I close the blinds and there's still lots of white space refusing to accept the gray matter from my brain. I'm on the third round of drops to take the pressure off. Preservatives, preservative free, although far from free in any other guise. When asked if the tier can be lowered to lower the cost, the insurance company gurus say, "No, no, a thousand times, no." Well, I exaggerate, it only seems a thousand. Maybe I refer to the number of over the counter tears I put into my eyes to soothe the cornea, or maybe it's the number of tears I shed in despair for my eyesight.

As we who are growing older disgracefully, have discovered, there must be a focus in our lives, or time forgets to march on, it just crawls along to some extraterrestrial beat. My focus has been my blog. When all else fails, I blog and life picks up the pace once again. I admit to a bit of self-indulgence. There are days when I can hit the computer with some discomfort, but I'm not always sure the discomfort is only in my eyes or perhaps also in the connection to my brain.

We recall the old song about the knee bone and its connection to the hip bone and so on down or up the line. Our discomfort or pain, as we might call it, could be anywhere, and we could decide that we don't want to add to our grief by forcing ourselves to do something, or anything, for that matter, and so we remove focus from our vocabulary - at least for the moment - and we plant our butts in our favorite chair and space out for a bit.

Okay for once in a while, but if you have learned, as have I, that a good conversation with oneself is very helpful and keeps you on the straight and narrow, you'll say the words that we all need to hear now and then. For me, it's "get up", "walk", "read", "write your blog". And a few other words that I prefer to keep to myself.

Get it? Pick your own words and be sure to have that conversation with yourself. What is your focus? Do you enjoy playing cards? Great, then do it. You had too much to eat and a little nap would be good, but it would interfere with your card game. There's always mañana and mañana, and no one will miss you, but they will, and it will mess up the game. Go, you lazy sluggard. Good friends and some fun, and you might win. Feel better after, don't you?

Me, too. Did my blog and it was no big deal. Eyes a little foggy? Yes, they are, but brain feels pretty good. I've been putting things off. Been having a little pity party for me. You know how that goes, but no one shows up and you might as well have saved the pity.

Forget the eyes. The ayes have it! The ayes always win - don't they? Aye, they do.

5. LET'S HEAR IT FOR GENERATION SPEAK

Is it some weird means of expression or are we speaking in some new form of code? Well, yes and no, depending on your point of view. I have made a critical and quite significant discovery, and along with the belief that all men are created equal - along with some women- I believe that all generations are not. The disparity among generations is overwhelming and that's why we need to find new ways to communicate.

Depending on the generation to which you belong, you will perceive the world in a particular way, and that way will belong to your generation only, despite protestations from those in or even outside of your group. Yes, perception is a generational thing and although sometimes I wish it were not, we all know that wishing does not make it so, regardless of our generational affiliation.

So, we, in the growing older disgracefully generation, look at those who have succeeded us, and try to explain that we have walked in their shoes- perhaps what seems like a long time ago- but they have not yet walked in ours and until they do, they cannot understand how we feel - impossible, no matter how hard they try.

It's a generational thing, we protest, but our words fall on deaf ears. We understand, they say, and of course they do not. In the simplest of words, you are not there until you are there, and could we make it any plainer than that? Oh my dear, I doubt it, but none are so deaf as those who will not hear.

I'm frustrated. In that long ago time when my parents said that I didn't understand, did I understand that I didn't understand, or was I stuck in the generational gap? I was. Was I? Oh yes, I'm sure I was.

6. WHERE HAVE ALL THE PEOPLE GONE?

Poignant words from Peter, Paul and Mary, but they were referring to flowers. No less poignant our words, only we refer to people. Where have they all gone, anyway? That question is a biggie and there's no simple answer, at least not in our book, and I'll bet your book has the same old pages as mine. In fact, that sentiment was the basis of a discussion that a friend and I had the other night. We decided that we who are growing older disgracefully have many more similarities than differences, only since we have pretty much stopped listening to one another, we obviously think that we're unique.

    For instance, we're all lonely at times- different times, varied times - but here it is, a paucity of people, contrasting with those times when we would have sold our souls to be given a moment's peace and quiet. You know, those, why don't they ever leave me alone moments. Remember that old saying about being wary of what you ask for etc. etc. etc.. I'm not an "I told you so" type, but I did tell you so, more times that I can recall.

Anyway, to get back on track, we decided that after a certain age, you get tired more easily, you lose the energy you used to have, something always hurts when you get out of bed in the morning, you always feel alone at some time or another and you forget things, things that you knew as well as the back of your hand, the same hand that ached when you got out of bed this morning. But - and this is important - you never talk about your feelings. Just about your pain, like your aching back or knees or neuropathies or whatever.

But what about if something happens and you need help and might become a burden? What about being nervous sometimes about driving, even though you still have your car? What about worrying about falling because everyone tells you that you could lose your balance, and that taking a tumble could change your life? What about the times when the phone doesn't ring and you know your family cares, but they have lives of their own? You have friends and you play cards and you eat lunch, but when you get up at night or you can't sleep, where's the voice that wants to know if you're all right?

That's when we ask where have all the people gone? We all do. We all ask, each and every one of us. We're not alone, and only we understand what is happening. We're in a very special club and you can't join till you're standing in our shoes. Hey, let's speak up. We're unique, but we're not alone. Sounds good to me. How about you?

7. A SON IS A SON

Till he takes him a wife. A daughter's a daughter for all of your life. Not absolutely true. A son is still yours, to be shared with another woman, a woman who sometimes forgets his beginning years when you were the sole caretaker. You were privy to his private parts and there were no raised eyebrows, and his early meals were just the way he liked them, and on time. Was everything perfect? No, of course not. Remember, a mother starts out as someone's wife and there's a steep learning curve between the two positions, but despite our perceived shortcomings, we seem to do well at mastering both. Until we become the daughters in law who will, in the natural order of progressions, wear the hats of wife, mother, and so on, ad infinitum or ad nauseam, if you prefer.

I'm still on the fence, I confess. Have been a daughter in law and a mother in law and thought I was exemplary in the first role but now I'm not so sure. My husband's mother went most everywhere with us, meaning my husband and children, especially after she was widowed, and she hardly was left to be on her own, but she's not around anymore. Exemplary does not seem to be something to strive for these days, be it kin by blood, or by statute. Busy is the buzz word, and as we who are growing older disgracefully have learned, the shortage of time is not experienced by ourselves, but mostly by those others in our lives who do not have any time on their hands - time for us, that is.

So what I have learned is that we live in a frenzied world, and that a daughter in law is not a daughter, and having started out as someone's daughter, we may remain in the daughter category, and mothers in law will not be mothers, after having worn the pseudo stigma of in law status. Therefore, when you get old and need the ministrations of a daughter, such ministrations will not be readily available without a genuine daughter to offer them.

There is no remedial solution to the absence of a daughter, at the time of life when most of us no longer have the equipment to be in production. Amen to that, I must say, thinking about additional nocturnal visits to the bathroom and the abdomens which refuse to stay in their place.

So, if there is no daughter, sons will sometimes rise to the occasion, but with wives who have supplanted daughters, beginnings will be ground into the dust and a son will remain the offspring who has taken a wife. A wife, a wife, is all lost to the wife? Not always. After all, a son is still a son.

8. YOU DON'T BRING ME FLOWERS

Seems like the last time I got flowers I was lying in a hospital bed, and the time before that I was going to my senior prom. Perhaps I exaggerate slightly, but truth to tell, I was never surrounded by romantic men. My first husband was never empty handed, but his taste ran more to pastrami than roses and far be it from me to minimize a pastrami sandwich on rye, but a rose is a rose is a rose -You get my drift?

We, who are growing older disgracefully, seem at times to be most sensitive to the sweetness of yesteryear. We remember gestures of sentiment that made us feel so special, and we yearn to experience those feelings once more.

Anyway, I guess I've made my point, that it's been a long time between horticultural offerings, and when the delivery men come to the lobby of my senior apartment complex, with a magnificent floral display, I admit to sometimes feeling a little sad and even a tad envious, at times. My neighbor and good friend's daughter, sent her a beautiful pot of tulips for Valentine's Day, but not having a daughter has lowered my expectations for the "girlie" things in life.

So, the most amazing thing happened to me last Sunday morning and it set me to thinking about lots of things. My neighbor from down the hall knocked on my door- I had just stepped out of the shower and was damply disheveled. She held out her arm, hand grasping a bunch of flowers and said that the flowers she was holding were from Church and were for me.

I stuck them into a vase filled with water and philodendra and spent the next few minutes admiring their beauty. They were more like wild flowers than flower shop display, but that was not important. Someone had given me flowers and I was such a woman again. Really, it takes so little for us to make one another happy. Why don't we do it more often?

To be more specific, why don't we take the time to find out what will please the other person or persons in our lives? If you'd said that to my husband, he would have said," why didn't she speak up? I would have gladly have also given her a pickle." If garlic be the food of love, then why did it take me so long to find out?

9. WHAT'S UP DOC?

Aside from an elevated opinion of yourself, what is up? Gosh, I've wanted to say that for a long time, but I've gotten timid in my old age, and I don't want to get you mad at me. We understand that you're a busy person and we have lots of time, but it wasn't always that way. Once upon a time we had real jobs and people came to us for advice and treated us with respect. Lots of things have changed, but the doctor/patient relationship seems to be the one that impacts us the most. And why not? You're the healer, the one person who seems to hold the key of life. Is that too much of a burden?

See, it's like this. Getting old is a part of the progression of life and there is no other option. Well there is, but we're not discussing extreme measures.

We who are getting older disgracefully, followed the rules when we were younger, and we put up with them because we were told that it would all come out right, at the end, but it has not. We're nearing the end and we want to be pleased with our life, we want some of that inner peace we hear so much about. You're the doctor, the healer, as I previously said, and we don't seem able to regard you as such.

Let's go back to the beginning of my lament. We know that many of our doctors have no patience with their patients (pun intended). Patients are noncompliant in many ways, ask inappropriate or too many questions, don't listen as carefully as they should and in general, are just a big nuisance. That may be true, but it goes with the territory. It's not so easy to listen when the ears are not fully functional and repetitious behavior is the result of a memory that plays tricks with our brains.

We need you and so many times you disappoint us. We are well aware that you are not The Almighty and that you are limited in what you can offer us. But, we are all human beings and we start out at the same place, and no matter where our footsteps take us, we all exit in the same way. So, like the song goes, "Try a Little Tenderness." It's not such a bad job. You could have been cutting the pastrami or maybe even "hold the pickles." Think about it. We do sometimes, when we sit and sit and wait for you. We don't mind the wait, it's what's waiting for us at the end of the rainbow, that hurts.

10. WHO FIXES YOUR INCOME?

We use that term all the time. I'm living on a fixed income, we say. Well of course we are. Almost all incomes are fixed. The important question is, who's doing the fixing?

If you were salaried, you pretty much got the same amount every month or week, as fixed by your employer. If you worked strictly on commission, your income may have varied from one pay period to the next, but even that might have been reasonably similar if you worked on some sort of draw arrangement. Let's go back to the source of your fixed income. The fallacy in using the term "fixed income" is an implication that you are suffering some sort of financial hardship and you may very well be, but we then go back to who is the fixer?

If you're on a pension, while it may be the same amount every payment, you may be getting a substantial figure, enough to keep you living reasonably well. After all, at this time in your life, you are assumedly not sending kids to college, feeding and clothing a family, and making capital purchases, and if you do the latter, it will most likely be based on savings, or sale of previous such purchases.

If you have income from investments and the like, you may be the fixer, having decided how much you need each month to live on. Although you may be desirous of more at times, you make the decision, bearing in mind that your assets have to last for a time that cannot be predetermined, unless you have the ability to foresee the future and if so, I want to hear from you. Now, please.

There is one source of income that is fixed by another party, and which cannot be influenced or changed by you, no matter what. I speak of Social Security, administered by the government and guided by a series of regulations. These rules determine the what, when and how our monthly payments will be distributed, and they are truly described as fixed. If you live strictly on social security payments, you are living on a fixed income. As you have learned, no amount of grumbling will affect the cost of living increase, and your opinion that you should have, and furthermore deserve, such an increase, will not make a difference.

So lets' bear in mind the various interpretations of the word "fixed." If you're the fixer, or even a former employer has done the fixing, you will get a stipulated amount, plus social security, of course. But when the social security administration, as advised by Congress, sends out your monthly check, and when that check is your only source of income, well, you get my drift. Maybe you were lucky and worked a lot, a lot, a lot, and got the maximum the government has to offer. Maybe not, and maybe, you'll think more carefully about whom you're electing, next time you step into the voting booth. Growing older disgracefully is learning at last, who is in charge.

11. JUST A SIMPLE FISH STORY

I find that living alone is even better when you have some other living creatures around. (No, in my book, mice and or rats, do not count). My dog is wonderful, of course, and when I moved in, I set up a fish tank - just six gallons - which is adequate for a small space and for small fish. Aye, and as the Bard would say, there's the rub. I bought two goldfish called Black Mollies, and because they are somewhat more expensive than plain old goldfish, I bought another goldfish called a "feeder" to test the water in the tank. Kind of like the tasters that Kings used to keep around, to make sure their food was free from poison.

Well, this little old taster just grew and grew and grew until he spanned the width of the tank. The other goldfish also grew - not to the degree of the taster - and everyone who came to visit commented on the humongous gold fish, who really cut a golden swath across the tank. After a while, the words of admiration turned to words of condemnation for me. How could I keep this poor fish in such a small tank? He must be truly miserable. Not as miserable as I, beginning to feel like a slum landlord, with my undersized tank and my oversized fish.

What was really becoming a problem was the inability of the small filter in this small tank to keep the tank clean. If you have ever had an aquarium and goldfish, you will know what I mean. Goldfish can eat prodigious amounts of food and are just as prolific in the amount of waste matter they generate. Despite constant water and filter changes, the fish lived in a smog-like environment.

The solution? A bigger tank. Ten gallons and a change from a hexagon to four large sides. I hoped the fish were happy because I was. I got up in the middle of the night and they were smiling. How do I know they were smiling? Simple, because they were no longer scowling. However, if they again seemed discontent, they would be replaced with living plants, and the tank would be called a terrarium. This should be a satisfactory arrangement, unless I accidentally planted some seeds from Jack's beanstalk. There's always the possibility of a turtle, one who would live forever and could be a heritage to my family. Who says there's nothing left to pass along?

Well of course, if there's a part one, there has to be a part two and sadly, here it is. Actually I shouldn't say sadly, because the ending of this story will not bring tears to your eyes. As we know, the best laid plans often go awry and one night the fish stopped smiling and within days they all succumbed to a condition which I was told by the fish store experts, is a result of overcrowding. Communal living is not for everyone. This time I would get it right. A new five gallon tank that looks bigger than it is, and is obviously made for a carefree bachelor.

This Black Molly goldfish, whom I assume is a he (and no one has proven me wrong) was the size of a penny, and now enormously spans the tank, keeps it meticulously clean, swims around what seems to be endlessly, darting in and out of the bubble wand and only seems to scowl, when friends comment on his solitary state. (my friends - I haven't met his). He's obviously very happy with his bachelor pad and as I said at the beginning of this fish tale, it's nice when you're alone, to have some other living creature around. So what am I? Chopped liver?

12. ADVICE WITH CONSENT

I have been giving a great deal of thought to what I am about to write. Because I have strong feelings, I think about my words sometimes before I go to sleep, and I think about them after some intense conversations that I wish had never taken place, and I have come to some conclusions.

We might need to pass a law: Unasked for advice is illegal and immoral, and should be subject to a fine based on the degree of irritation which the unwilling recipient experiences. Now let us be clear. I have nothing against seeking out advice. At times, I have received some amazing advice, but the advice has been sought out by me and most often based on what I perceive to be the expertise of the person with whom I consult.

The key words there being "sought out." Admittedly, like so many of us who are growing older disgracefully, I can be a stubborn cuss, and am somewhat weary of people who obviously think they can live our lives better than we. Maybe they're right, but since, in theory at least, we are all created equal, I demand my constitutional right to blunder my way through life, unassisted, until on bended knee or merely with head bowed, I beg for help.

The problem with unasked for advice - aside from its being unasked for - is the source from which it springs. With access to myriad TV gurus and the Internet, many of us are under the impression that we have all learned all there is to know about everything, and some of us feel a strong need to share. My answer to them is "resist."

Many of us feel a heartfelt desire to help others, and what better way is there than to provide our fellow man or woman with advice that will enrich their lives, and we have the words to do it. But do we? Let's use quitting smoking, as an example. We all know that smoking is a bad thing and aside from offering immediate pleasure, has long range, very deleterious effects, but do we all know how to stop? Do we all know how hard it is? Even if we have done it, we are all different and what works for one may not work for all. I was a smoker, and if you ask me how I quit, I would gladly tell you, with the caveat that because it worked for me, there is no guarantee that it will work for you.

    I have to be honest. I gave more advice when I was younger, and I'm sure most of it was unasked for, but I knew more when I was younger, than I do now. How is that possible? Is my brain shrinking? No, I don't think so. I believe my ego is. Growing up, it was hard to admit that so many knew more than I. Now I know that many do, and what's more important, it doesn't matter. Want some advice? Beg me.

13. TIME ON OUR HANDS

One of the most striking things that occurred when I entered grouchland, was having more time than I'd had for years, but always feeling rushed because I thought I didn't have enough. After a lifetime of having worked eight hour plus days, I would be entering la la land unless I addressed this issue.

All of a sudden I could do whatever I wanted, whenever I wanted, and there were no demands on my time except for the occasional visit to a doctor. I could stay up all night and I just might, in spite of trying to sleep, because I had an unexpected doze-off during the day, or had done nothing more strenuous than exercise my facial muscles at mealtimes.

In the beginning, such great freedom is a heady

thing. I stayed up late, watching a movie or a TV show that kept me up until the single digits, but it really didn't matter. The next morning, because my little dog is ravenously hungry by 7AM, I would get up, feed her, let her out and go back to bed, sometimes sleeping until as late as 10 or 11 AM. After getting up, I would exercise for half an hour, then have breakfast at the time I was accustomed to having lunch. It does make for a short morning. In fact, it makes for a very short day, which feels somewhat aimless at times.

I have nothing against leisure. You know how we're always talking about someday when we have time, well someday is here and I have time, and I am learning that a commodity has value in inverse proportion to its availability. Scarcity imparts a move up the scale for everything, and I need to move time from the plus to the minus column. I need to move time from being on my hands to being in my hands and how am I going to do that?

I need to add something to my life. I need to move my excess time from the overflowing basket I am carrying, to the basket that seems never to be full. I need to add a special word to my life and for me that word seems to be *focus*. Focus, direction, meaning, purpose – call it what you like. I prefer focus because one definition says, "focus is the concentration of attention or energy on one thing." And I get to choose the thing. I can take all of my time or little of my time or whatever chunk of time appeals to me, and direct it to wherever I want. I can decide that this is the time to read all the great books I have never read, or maybe even write a few that have been rattling around in my brain. Maybe I just want to plop myself in my favorite rocker for hours at a time and think amazing thoughts, or clear out my brain and don't think at all, as if being in a perpetual state of meditation.

Whatever I decide, I have made a conscious decision. My life is not aimless. I know the direction I'm going and it's completely acceptable to me. If I decide to just sleep late every day there's nothing wrong with that, if *I* think there's nothing wrong with that.

This is the time of life when I need answer only to myself and if I'm pleased with the answers I get, then maybe I have reached the state of equanimity I may have been searching for all of my life.

Kind of a neat goal, isn't it, just being content. Some of us never achieve that goal and isn't it nice that I not only have time on my hands, it's my time and it's also in my hands. I have to remember that someday means now and the future might be here, so if I'm going to kick up my heels, the time for orange hair has arrived or would I look better in blue? What have you been putting off?

14. A VOTE IS A TERRIBLE THING TO WASTE

Must be true because lately, whenever my phone rings, there's a voice on the other end begging me to give my vote to the candidate of his/her choice. Soliciting of any kind is a bottom of the pile job, and having been in that unenviable position once or twice, way back when, I tend to be more tolerant than I would be ordinarily and usually forgo the grand slam.

Politics aside, I'm a Floridian now, and in the past, for example, I recall hearing most frequently from the supporters of David Jolly and Alex Sink. I had decided that their futures would be more sanguine with a change of name. I mean, after all, who wants to think about Sink or swim or the folly in not having voted for Jolly. Movie stars change their names all the time and it seems only to have enhanced their careers.

Many calls come from as far away as Texas or Pennsylvania, so I guess it must be party unity that brings support to candidates in Florida, and also why the calls always seem to come at some inconvenient time, like when I'm in the loo or the shower. Not their fault, but when you're the recipient, you get pretty prickly about things.

If you really want my vote, make sure your candidate has sworn to keep his/her cotton pickin' hands off my social security, unless he/she has found some miraculous way to restore the former value to the COLA affecting my social security check. Absent that, I have no interest in any candidate regardless of his pre-election promises.

Once I reached the voting age, I have always voted. I consider a vote a sacred obligation and a privilege, as well. I don't need a reminder and I don't appreciate being coerced into voting for some candidate of whose last name I do not approve. And so, I shall write in the name of my candidate of choice. Some sturdy names like Washington, Jefferson, Roosevelt or Lincoln. You know, names that don't actually move a mountain but sure do look good on the face of it.

15. KICKING THE HABIT

Old habits die hard - Old habits are like old shoes. They don't pinch anymore, but sometimes when we walk on pebbles or in the rain, we feel a twinge here and there and we know there's moisture inside as well as out. But what the heck - we're used to them and starting over is such a pain. So, being the creatures of habit that we are, we try to keep on with the same old behavior that has become a no brainer.

When I've tried to analyze what it is about a habit that makes it so steadfast, it seems to be closely related with my zone of comfort. The thing about habits is that they can be good or bad and thereby hangs the rub. We want to keep our good habits. For instance, brushing our teeth in the morning is essential, or so we've been told by Dr. Gums, and we wouldn't want to have a debate with ourselves every day - to brush or not to brush. It, being a habit, we automatically brush and that's a good thing.

So, when to kick and how to kick and how to decide if it's a habit we even want to kick. First we have to categorize. Good, bad or pain in the butt before it became attached to our psyche? Another example. Getting undressed at night and immediately hanging up our clothes before going to sleep, or leaving garments where they fall as we remove them from our frames, and just stepping around then in the morning, especially if here's no one to complain. I confess, I'm a compulsive hanger upper and on the rare occasions when having imbibed a bit more than appropriate, I just drop everything to the floor, but the moment I awake, I set about cleaning house. At times, habits such as these can be annoying, but only on a case by case basis.

However, there is one habit that almost universally can be classified as bad, and that is the habit that I dropped many years ago. and whose dropping caused me more emotional pain than anything I have done before or since. The SMOKE QUIT! Yes, I did it and went cold turkey and I think that's the best thing I've done for my life, at least in the opinion of every doctor I have seen since the quit, and as I am among those who are growing older disgracefully, that's a lot of doctors.

My dog, Daisy, who from time to time, looks over my shoulder as I write, understands about being a creature of habit. Just move something out of its place and she almost loses her woofer. I understand. Losing your woofer is most definitely something to bark about. Woof, woof !!

16. KERMIT, KERMIT, WHERE IS MY PERMIT?

If you have a handicapped parking permit and you forget to hang it in the window when you exit your car, you could find yourself up the creek without a paddle. Or at least it might feel that way. And so I have written myself a little ditty and I am searching for a little green frog to hang in my window as my memory jogger, because I don't want to mess with the police again.

You see, before I was citationed, I parked my car in the main library parking lot, the library where I volunteer for two to three hours every Thursday, loaded with a full bag of books from my favorite candy store. In my haste to improve my tardiness record, I move quickly, at dinosaur's pace, from the car to the building and yes, due to my inability to multitask, I forget to hang my permit. Along comes the Gendarme -maybe it's a slow day and there aren't many violators - and whoops, there's a car in a handicapped space and there's no permit hanging against the windshield.

So I finish my stint in the library and there's something tucked against the windshield and if it were an ad, all the cars would have one but no, just me, and it's a citation. $255 fine and my heart jumps out of my chest. I know I can't pay it, so I know I must dispute it, but it's such a process. In addition, whoever issued the citation, accused me of parking my car in lot 10 at City Hall and not in the parking lot at the public library.

Everything has to be copied and sent to the DMV as proof of having a permit. First you phone and protest the incorrectness of the parking lot, and you are not accused of nitpicking in so many words, but that's the general idea. After all, an overloaded police department can't be expected to get everything right. So you send a copy of everything requested and you better get everything right - and then you wait. You call the DMV for the next 4 weeks and you're told it's under review. What are they reviewing? Your stupidity or your inability to multitask? Also, you are only allowed to have this memory lapse once a year, so you'd better never again forget to hang your permit in the window.

At last the letter comes. I have been forgiven and the citation is rescinded. I put the permit on the passenger seat because tucking it into the glove compartment is too risky. As they say, out of sight out of mind. I drive over to a toy store to find a little frog, small enough not to block my view, and I hang him from my mirror. I name the keeper of my permit, Kermit, and now I just have to hope that I remember why Kermit is hanging from my mirror. And that Kermit rhymes with permit. Oh, and that the DMV is not intolerant of memory loss. At least not more than one time a year.

17. LET'S HEAR IT LIKE IT IS

Are you as fed up as we are with words from 50 year olds telling us how it feels to be 85? Give us a break, or at least let us hear from folks who are walking in our orthopedic shoes. Shoes, which, by the way, create a difference in perspective from sheer heel height alone. After all, 4-6 inches above the sidewalk has to affect the way we are grounded.

So where are all the oldsters who should be growing older disgracefully by letting the world know how we feel? The next time you mention to one of your offspring, how tired you are, and they assert that they know exactly how you feel, try to discover how they know. If they're not impressed with your owning 35 more years of wear and tear than they, try comparing yourself to an old car with lots more mileage than a new vehicle. That's a concept that nearly everyone can grasp.

Did you believe, when you saw Grandma doze off in front of the TV, at 3 in the afternoon, that you would be that same Granny, getting forty winks during the day, sitting up in a chair. Don't understand why it happens. Even after a good night's sleep the body seems to crave a little jolt of zzzs to recharge the battery.

You used to be an exercise junkie - every other AM before work, a quick session at the gym and maybe a little jog on the weekend. Now you take an occasional walk around the complex where you live, make a trip by car to the supermarket, then home again, home again, and when did those bundles of groceries get so heavy? Did you realize how much you had bought? Just one solitary bottle of juice. Nothing like the soda and beer you used to carry. In your sit and be fit class you do lift some 1 lb weights, but when you did workouts with Jane Fonda, the weights were more like 7 - 10 lbs. Sometimes.

What about all those wonderful plans you make and break? Going to go through all the old papers you've been meaning to clear out and throw away? You start and then you get involved in some TV show you've started to watch and what's the hurry, anyway? There's always tomorrow when you're not so worn out. The drive and motivation you used to have seems to have gone into hibernation. In fact, growing towards triple digits might be termed hibernation in situ. Nothing phenomenal is going to develop. Actually, maintenance, not development, is the order of the day. Not such a bad thing. Even type A personalities say enough already, when the time is right. And old type A's always know when it's right.

18. KIND: A FORGOTTEN FOUR LETTER WORD?

My sons were often chastised, as they were growing up, for overuse of certain four letter words, words which I hope have since been dropped from their vocabulary, and if not, they are no longer used in my hearing. But with what have these words been replaced? Not "love" or most certainly, "kind", because there don't appear to be a surfeit of them there words around. At least not in practice, so maybe they're being reserved for spelling bees. Easy to spell. A little more difficult to define or use as an adjective, modifying behavior.

More and more frequently I have long conversations with myself and my dog, Daisy (and to anyone else who will listen) asking why we can't be kind to one another. Is it easier to be cruel? A conundrum, it is, and does that mean it offers no solution, at best? I have become a devotee of the animal channels on TV, trying to get an insight into animal behavior and thereby getting some insight into the behavior of my two legged peers. In particular, the residents of the senior complex where I live, those who are growing older disgracefully, by adhering to the Golden Rule.

But are they? Are they doing unto others what they would have others etc. etc. etc.? Just a few days ago, an act of such mean spirited unkindness was perpetrated by an unknown coward, desecrating a bill board display, for no apparent reason, and I, for one, am left feeling sad and personally despoiled. This is an act of cruelty that I see repeated in many different guises at varying times and in many different degrees, but that is not the only issue.

Another long interior monologue with myself. We have lived a long life, experiencing good and bad and we are still blessed with choice. Amazing to have choice when there are so many aging persons around us with no choice, just happy to have a roof over their heads and accompanying food. Let's take "kind" out of moth balls. Let's use it, do it, say it, make it so much a part of ourselves that we become tongue tied without it. And do me a favor. If I seem to forget, just remind me. That would be the kindest act of all.

19. THE PECKING ORDER

I never gave much thought to the existence of a pecking order, until I became one of those folks who are growing older disgracefully. I recognize how pervasive the pecking order is, in particular, where the generations coexist and seniors are in the minority, and now, it has become a part of my consciousness.

For example, I registered on Face book - as I register at many other sites - just because they're free and I can. Unlike my grandchildren and myriad friends, I never change my profile picture. Why would I? I was three years younger and I'm just about the only one who looks at it, anyway. Most of my peers are not computer aficionados, their notebooks are frames for their photographs, and their cell phones are mainly for texting. Besides, my friends at my senior complex are happy to tell me how they feel, if I ask them…more graphically and in greater detail than they ever could on Face book.

My visits to Face book are occasioned by an email informing me that I have a notification, frequently pertaining to people I have never met. As for the ones I have met, I'm not always sure that they have met me. Or at the least, remember me. I use that invitation to visit Face book as an opportunity to become, at least pictorially, reacquainted with my grandchildren, especially the ones who grew up with me, before our geographical distancing. I never visit Face book to chronicle my fascinating or more often, boring life, at least in the eyes of those who have succeeded me.

I'm delighted to see the changing profile pictures of my granddaughter and some of the insightful comments about life in general, but I wonder if I need a formal application to be included, or at least get honorable mention, as a friend of the family. After a visit to Florida, the highlight of her visit was a photo of her and a dolphin. Shows good taste, anyway. Dolphins are so smart. I like Ahi Tuna and so does my grandson, so maybe there's a raw fish connection between me and the dolphins and my grandson and by extension, the rest of the family.

What has all the above to do with pecking

orders? My opinion is that Face book strongly reinforces the belief that grandparents are the lowest persons in the pecking order of the family. In fact, when former United States President, Bill Clinton, began a discussion with former United States President George Bush, pertaining to Bush's role as a grandparent, George Bush defined a grandparent as the lowest person in the pecking order of the family. Amazing, two men who didn't fall off a turnip truck in their former lives, but who held the position which belongs to the most powerful person in this country, and they have been, or will consider themselves, relegated to the bottom of the family pecking order.

Like Tina Turner, who asked what's love got to do with it? I paraphrase and ask what's age got to do with it? Plenty, and that's the problem. We are a civilization which is hung up on numbers. Social Security used to be the identifier, but now, in addition, you're asked for your birth year, which you offer sotto voce, the way you used to mumble your weight at weight watchers.

I admit I do play the age card when the lines are very long, and someone offers to let me cut in. Don't get to play that card very often in a state where there's so much white hair and lots of accompanying wrinkles. However, when I'm out in the world and people can only guess at my age, and it's every woman for herself, I do as I've done all of my life. I cope. In fact, I sometimes more than cope, because it's the only option in town.

However, the pecking order comes into play when I am in the rightful place in which my family places me. I can't find my keys. Understandable. I am old and my memory has been seriously eroded. I have to make a decision to change my health plan. Someone needs to step up to the plate. I was a Health Care Executive for 25 years, but that was before my apparent lobotomy. As for anything wireless? Inappropriate time of birth. When it comes to uploading and downloading? Hopeless. I don't really want to play with your toys, anyway. You can wear your Google glasses but you still won't be able to decipher my cursive correspondence. So there! Don't know much about androids, but dinosaurs were pretty exciting once upon a time. Still - just remember extinction!

20. MOTHER'S DAY -- A COMMERCIAL HOLIDAY?

The kids were growing up and away from observing holidays like Mother's Day, but that's probably because Daddy was the one who used to make the fuss, and take everyone out to eat at some special restaurant. This was not the day for mom to cook. These days I've learned not to be too inquisitive, but I confess to a bit of curiosity. Is mother's day a special time for my daughters in law, or has that also gone the way of real letters and special cards?

I see flower deliveries on the front desk of the lobby, in the complex where I live. To be honest, I was the recipient of flowers one Mother's Day, from my darling dog, Daisy, by way of a friend, who is growing older disgracefully, as am I, My friend and I spent a wonderful week together and she will foster Daisy, if I am given early retirement to my cabin in the sky.

I always sent my mother a card, even when we were apart, but that probably wasn't enough, and is on my list of do overs, should I get the chance. My mother-in-law, who lived nearby, was given a celebratory day, alongside me.

Since I have concluded that growing older is a reversal of the steps taken when we are growing up, I understand why we are so affected by those around us. It's like being back in school, where your ranking was so important. Those of us who are not taken out on Mother's Day, sit together at what I have characterized as the orphan's table, so that we don't feel alone.

I hate to admit to being so mean spirited, but all the showing around of cards proclaiming love and all that jazz, does make me wish that I had more dogs. Also sad for the son who is no longer here and who I always miss, and who didn't consider Mother's Day a commercial holiday. He's also on my list of do overs.

Mother's Day. Makes me question my skills as a mother and also makes me question what I could have done or should have been. For me, the longer I live, the longer my list of do-overs gets. It's okay.

They're part of the human condition. As am I.
Happy Mother's Day.   ou, too, Hallmark!

21. IF ONLY………

As the New Year begins and nostalgia raises its pervasive head, we think of all the things we might have done and didn't, and wonder why or why not. Not so much the life changing events, but the trivial or even silly things that we think we can no longer do.

For instance - as I watched an awards show the other night - I suddenly realized that even when I could afford them, I never owned a pair of Manolo Blahnik shoes. Even if Santa had left a pair of Manolos (as we in the know, refer to them) under the tree, I could have bronzed them, as we did our offsprings' baby shoes, or built an alter on which to display them, but never, never could I have attempted to squeeze my calloused, crooked toes onto the leather pedestals that proclaim to the fashionistas of the world, that I can walk the walk like the best. As opposed to the present time when I am happy just to walk like the rest.

A friend - one of those who like me are attempting to grow older disgracefully- just retired to Colorado, and she invited me to spend some time with her. She is only fully alive when she has a pair of skis attached to her feet and she offered to give me lessons. My first attempt on skis was a slope in Vermont many years ago. It was not for beginners, but when the 5 year olds were off and running, or at least standing, I decided that skiing was not for me. I regret that decision because unlike many other sports, there seems to be no age related cut off. However, since I just completed a course in balance training, and now put falling and subsequent breakage on the top of my avoidance list, skis, like Manolos, are not coming out of the closet.

It appears that my "if onlys" have a greater relationship to my lower limbs than to what rests above my neck. I came to this conclusion when I recalled that at one long ago time in my life, I thought I might want to run. We lived in a state that sponsored yearly marathons, which I could view from my apartment window. The energy was so strong it seemed to fill the air and I experienced it as something of which I wanted to be a part. However, like so many of the thoughts which trickle in and out of our minds, it was never put into action until one day the realization came to me that the distance from my window to the marathon, was more than eighteen stories, it was more like a universe apart.

    As I struggle to walk on my treadmill, gasping slightly on some days, and wondering on other days, which part of my body will be the first to surrender, I think of how lucky I am to have a few trivial 'if onlys' and no serious regrets. Besides, I'm too preoccupied with 'what ifs,' to be bothered with anything else.

22. THE INFORMERS

Sounds like a remake of an old movie, or a TV series featuring Elliot Ness and his cohorts. Maybe so, but our informers are not criminals, they're residents of senior complexes, who've never learned to fight their own battles and who go to "mommy," aka the manager, whenever their fellow residents are "naughty" to them.

Some of us oldsters have lived in apartment houses for much of our lives and we have long ago learned that shared spaces are not always idyllic- in fact, if you never learned about give and take, well - it's about time you did. The way it works is this way. For instance, I make noise and your make noise and we find a way to live with it. Like if you have a dog and I have a dog and they both bark - well that's what dogs do . Get a bird if you would rather have tweets, and maybe you can convince your neighbors, that they're also for the birds.

What inspired this whole tirade - if that's what this is - is a story told to me by a friend, who also lives in a senior complex, and who broke what was apparently a cardinal rule and was reported to the management. The rule, which is not on a wall, in a book or even in a lease, proscribes the wearing of night apparel in the public halls. According to this friend, she found herself in desperate straits one morning at 2 A.M. when she realized she needed to wash a pair of pants, part of an outfit she was planning to wear to a party the following day. Assuming that no one would be in the hall at that time, she hurried out in her night gown to the laundry room. But lo and behold, she met the "scold" from the floor, a woman who obviously noted her inappropriate attire and who, on the following day reported her to the manager

She (my friend) was summoned to the office of the manager, who recounted the incident and provided a stern admonishment and 2 chocolate chip cookies with apologies for being out of doughnuts.

Kudos for the manager and cuckoos for the resident. If we who are growing older disgracefully want to spread our wings and fly, so be it. Show and tell is fine, but I'm gonna tell is mean, and this close to

Evelyn Marder Levin

the pearly gates, who wants to be mean?

23. HURRY UP AND SLOW DOWN

I'm in no rush to get off the telephone, unless I have an appointment with a doctor or plans for lunch, and that doesn't happen very often. When I'm in the midst of a conversation, I hear the sound of a ring or a buzz of some sort, and I know that another call is waiting, but that's okay. For most of the world, the ring a ding or buzz or whatever sound is their interrupter - because that is what most phone calls are - I forget, because I do not have an interrupter, I have a connector. That beautiful sound which floats into my ears means that I will have a real conversation and how nice that is.

Someone is going to connect with me and if I am lucky and have been intermittently napping in front of the TV, I will interact with another person. We will exchange ideas, thoughts or maybe just gossip and I will again appreciate how the spoken word fills up space so deliciously. Oh I'm so delighted I do not text! That's because I refused to learn to type when I was young, since proper young ladies learned to type so that they could - if all else failed - become someone's secretary, and type and bring the morning coffee. I did not want to do any of those things and did not add typing to my skills. I could tell my younger friends that texting means they are typists, using a rather shorthanded form of the alphabet, but typing, none the less. Of course they run circles around me at the computer and the cell phone, but it's nice to know some of the old time skills are still around.

But back to the phone and its connections. Sometimes, I hear in the voice at the other end, a soupcon of impatience that is telling me my time is up or rather their time is up, and we have to cut the cord. There is no cord, but we have to cut something, and I am reminded of a doctor who stands at the door with his hand on the knob at the end of our session, another example of hurry up and slow down and you know which is which.

I watch people at the elevator, ire rising as the elevator does not and I wonder at their impatience. We who are growing older disgracefully, have learned that time is a commodity we have in abundance, and yet we are greedy at having to spend it. If truth be told, I am hardly ever in a rush. There are chores I must do daily - eye drops, pills, feed my dog and my fish - but then, extravagantly, I can spread my minutes wherever I wish. How decadent I have become. Thinking and day dreaming, what luxuries they are! People chafe at getting old and make negative comments, but we know the good stuff.

    All my life I was in a hurry. Time was in a short supply. But now, I'll put on my music or watch a DVD and I've forgotten how it feels to be in a hurry. I'm too busy slowing down, slowing down, slowing down. Oh, it feels so good. Wish you had more time?

24. SHOOT THE MESSENGER, PLEASE!

"We become what we behold." Marshal McLuhan said in 1964, and to which I would add, we become what we are told to be.

Before the pervasiveness of the media, in particular television, we put our faith in journalism, which at one time referred almost exclusively to the written word. "Extra, extra! Read all about it!" The newsboys, hawking their papers on the street, would cry out the headlines of the day from the newspaper for which they worked.

We understood that the large, bold type on the front page related to the major story of the day-major in the opinion of the publisher of the newspaper. Okay. We could read it or not as we chose, and could discuss the story with family or friends, if sufficiently interested. We were not analysts or critics and might base our beliefs on what we considered to be solid evidence or maybe just on who had the kindest face. Simplistic? Perhaps, but we were all thinking machines in those days- some more rusty and ineffectual than others - but good, bad or indifferent, we put the little gray cells to work (as detective Poirot would have said) and the gray cells were a reflection of our own beliefs.

Flash forward to the new world, the world where one picture is worth a thousand words, but we get not only the picture, we also get the thousand words. We now have the bearer of dispatches (Job 1:14,) also called the messenger, from the Greek, angelos, and synonymously in English, the intelligencer. I take issue with the derivations of the word, messenger. The individuals who have taken it upon themselves to pre-chew and digest the information which is presented to us electronically, and who then, bird like, push into our mouths what they think we need to know, in whatever form they think we can absorb, are not angels - they are not sent from on high to inform us, unless on high refers to the political machinations of management - they are sent to bedevil us, to confuse us and to influence us and act as thought police who tell us how to interpret what we see and hear.

Who are these messengers, these intelligencers, these gurus who have the temerity to call themselves analysts and interpreters and who often are without credentials, save having been serendipitously attached to some news media by a fortuitous event?

I can observe a political convention or listen to a speech without benefit of ad nauseam analysis more based on opinion than on fact. I read prodigiously, as do many of us who are growing older disgracefully and we don't wait breathlessly for a TV commentator to tell us whether we liked, agreed with or disagreed with what was said. We don't want to watch an event which is being televised and for which the armchair analysts arbitrarily pick out what we may watch.

We resent having political commentary take place while we are trying to listen to a speech which we don't consider minor and which the analysts do, and so we must surf the channels to find someone who respects our right to choose. A hint to our fellow sufferers - public broadcast stations are usually more respectful of their viewer's preferences.

We want to know what's going on in the world. Report the news, televise the speeches, don't be decision makers, just be the reporters that you are meant to be. Most of us don't want information to be selectively revealed to us - be straight with us, or we may be tempted to deal with messengers, in the way did monarchs of old, when confronted with bearers of unpleasant news.

25. WHEN IS ENOUGH, ENOUGH?

As I gravitate towards those who are most often categorized as needy, I am no longer part of the greedy. My financial resources have been downsized, and my chief source of income is social security. I have learned that what I want, is only relevant when accompanied by phrases such as what I need.

Amazingly, as what I wanted seemed to shrink, what I needed was also reduced. I wondered, can really wealthy people with 3 or 4 homes, manage with only 1 or 2 if the need arises, when such a choice is purposefully made? Shopping, which had been a chief source of recreation for me, had become rather a bore, but I questioned if that was due to cranial development, or just a slide towards less disposable income?

As I looked around, I noticed I wasn't the only one in the supermarket with a near empty cart. I remembered when I could spend $100 in 10 minutes and now it takes me 100 minutes to spend $10. That was O.K. It wasn't until I encountered a true case of greed, where I live, that I became disturbed by how pervasive it is.

I sold a piece of my jewelry to an antique dealer, so that I could have a little money to buy some holiday gifts for the family. Unfortunately, the buyer left off my apartment number and her check was put into the mailbox of a woman with a similar name - not the same - just somewhat similar. The second misfortune was the greedy son-in-law of the woman who owned the mailbox. I won't use his real name - we'll just call him mister greed.

When I complained about not receiving the check, the dealer told me that it had gone to the wrong mailbox. The dealer's name was on the check and mister greed called her and said that though the names were somewhat different, it must belong to his mother-in-law, and she had just had a birthday party to celebrate a major birthday. Sixty people at a posh restaurant, open bar and individual menu choice - and so the check must be a gift for her, and he wouldn't hand the check over to me. By the time it was all sorted out - I had to bring in the police - and mister greed returned the check to me - 2 weeks had passed and it was too late for me to shop.

    For mister greed, enough is obviously never enough. Many of us who are growing older disgracefully, are making the transition from too much to not enough. What a difficult time to make such a discovery. At least, we are somewhat fortunate. We didn't grow up in the age of the I-phone and the I-Pad, and so we have learned that a little deprivation is not such a big deal- so long as we can afford a not so smart cell phone and one that is text enabled. Texting-the cool communication du jour! Too cool? Too much or maybe just enough?

26. BONE LOSS, NOT RETIREMENT, DIMINISHES

Last night I went to a party.
"What do you do?" I was asked.
"Nothing. I'm retired".
"Oh?"
That was a really dumb answer. I help keep the local library open by volunteering. In case you hadn't noticed, most libraries have had to cut their hours and it's old dames like me who fill in the bare spots left by staff layoffs, and we do it without affecting the budget. Our only reward is giving back to the community that kept us reading for so many years. Well, okay, let's be honest. Having first crack at all the new books and loading up on DVD's for the week - what I refer to as my weekly fix - ain't just chopped

liver.

So I'm not making any money, but I'm helping to save a little here and there, and in our nation's present financial crunch that's no small thing, multiplied by thousands of gray heads like mine. Actually, I probably owe the library, because the exercise to my brain is keeping the little gray cells active and maybe even multiplying.

I also volunteer with my little dog, Daisy, at some local nursing homes in my community. If you could see the smiles on the residents' faces when Daisy gives one of her juicy kisses, you'd smile, too, and remember one of these days you're going to get old and maybe lonely sometimes as well, and won't it be nice to have some adorable little dog slobbering over your face and making you feel loved? If you say no, you're just an old curmudgeon and we'll tell Daisy to save her kisses for someone more deserving.

I have lots more time to volunteer and I was considering being an usher at the local concert hall. I wasn't intimidated by having to stand for three hours, but that many hours without a bathroom break was too awful to even contemplate. Besides, I was apparently the only one who wanted to hear some of the concerts or see the shows. Everyone else was there purely to give back to the community and would have worked with plugs in their ears and blindfolded, if feasible. I guess I'm an old curmudgeon at times when I forget about the greater good.

I used to feel inadequate because I'm just a volunteer. Not getting paid for work means, in the minds of many, that it is somehow less important, less necessary. I know that's not so, although to be perfectly honest, if there were sufficient funds to pay for some of the freebies I'm doing, I would say bring it on. Living on a fixed income, there are not too many splurges, but once in a while you'd like to indulge in the national pastime and shop for something other than blood pressure or cholesterol medications, and maybe buy a pair of outrageous earrings that would be more suitable for your granddaughter.

I allow myself to be diminished, when others, including my offspring, imply that unpaid work is not really work, and while they struggle to put food on the table, I just sit back and bask in my social security payments, payments which took countless years to accumulate. Besides, while the younger folk are haunted by fears of job loss, we old folk worry about social security funds being raided to pay down the national debt. Being homeless is very bad, but homeless and old is having to relearn where all the public toilets are.

I grew up without a cell phone, a TV set and a

computer, but my family had a radio and we sat around, listening to it, every Sunday night. We oldsters should be very proud of ourselves in this century of galloping technology. We have mastered things that we didn't cut our teeth on in school, despite our being classified as dinosaurs. I don't mind. Unlike the dinosaurs, I refuse to fade away into extinction. I have lots to squeeze into whatever years remain and I intend to do it disgracefully. I hope there are lots of others out there who will do the same. Any ideas? Put on your thinking caps and flex your muscles. Me, Tyrannosaurus Rex.

27. WHERE'S THE EQUALITY?

I don't understand. More and more often I confront people who regard the ability to do something with one's hands, as superior to that which is achieved by brainpower. Regretfully, I use the word superior, when I want to say, different but equal, and yet I cannot, in the face of what I see as wrong headedness, on the part of so many people

Fortunately, this belief is not held across the board by the entire world, but unfortunately, depending on the surrounding community, beliefs may vary. For instance, in the academic community, there is no such thing as too much education or over development of the brain. In fact, the greater the number of degrees, the greater the respect for the individual, and this before inclusion of books authored, or papers written, or speeches given etc.. In further fact, skills other than those acquired by the various degrees, are often prevalent in these same people. Forgive my seeming repetition, but these same people are most frequently the ones who respect the skills and abilities of people who are competent in any way.

But, to return to my confusion regarding the varying abilities of different people, I must reiterate that I don't understand. Is someone who has driven a truck across the country all of his or her life, more accomplished than some other one who has studied for many years and learned how to construct the truck, which will be used to cross the country? Is the doer more important than the planner? Do we have to feel someone's muscle to respect their strength, and do we have to see a brain scan to respect what a person is capable of creating?

I live in a senior complex and I wonder, as a part of those who are growing older disgracefully, what are the acceptable terms of what is considered important and worthy of respect. A poem is only words on a page, but a wreath can have flowers and ribbons and seem to have taken hours to assemble. Is it not possible that the poet who created the poem also spent hours assembling the words from which that poem is created? Do we have to touch and actually feel a creation in order for it to be validated? Can we only respect that which we fully comprehend and which we might possibly regard as something we could possibly accomplish? In other words, if I don't play golf, what meaning can the skills of the man who is considered the greatest golfer in the world, have to me?

And so I respectfully ask, where is the equality? If beauty is in the eye of the beholder, is value in the brain of just one singular creature? No, we all have the ability to see, to appreciate, to respect. Please, let us see in each human being the special qualities that have been given to all. Let us open our minds and see and see and see. Can you see?

28. GROW OLD ALONG WITH ME, THE REST IS YET TO BE

Growing older is not a disease or a condition. It's a process which everyone has to go through unless you die young, of course. So you hot young babe, who looks at me with disdain, wondering if I forgot to iron my neck this morning, just bear in mind that your neck will wrinkle and sag just like mine. "Never," you say, "I'll go plastic." Go ahead. Have 1 or have 101, but sooner or later your body will catch up with you and you'll find yourself being given a seat on the bus, or getting an offer to have your groceries carried out to your car, or being addressed as "ma'am".

All of which you'll be grateful for, because you will have learned that aging is inevitable and the preferred option. The golden years. Ahh, if only they would increase in value similar to the way that gold has risen in the past several years. But the golden years seem tarnished at times, and I believe that's often due to our level of expectations. What was adorable in infancy - diapers, for example- is far from adorable in old age but let's face it, folks, it can happen across the board and we have to be grateful for what we avoid, bearing in mind that it all can be part of the process. The process - the process - the process.

That doesn't mean we have to succumb to a lesser ability to do things. As we discover in life to pick and choose our battles, so we must discover when we can push ourselves, and when we must ask for help. I have pain in my body so I can be crotchety and nasty and besides I am old and old people are different from other people. No, no and no. You haven't been paying attention. Old people are just babies with a hell of a lot of years added on. My cousin is 85 and she refuses to reveal her age. She claims to be 70 and no one doubts her. What does that mean? No one is rude enough to tell her that she looks old for 70, because she does. Why does it matter, anyway?

Our society has conditioned us to cringe when we old folks mention our ages. We have to get past that. I live in a senior complex where no one can be under 55, but most are over 70, and here, age is a badge of honor, especially if you're 90 and still do the meringue, or talk on the phone and drive, which further proves that age and wisdom don't go hand in hand.

Do I sometimes reflect back on what was and what I was? Absolutely. I'm human and I admit to all the frailties therein. But I had an interesting moment last week. I had been to see my cardiologist - from 75 on, everyone has a cardiologist - and he expressed himself as pleased with my general condition. I stood waiting for the elevator, thinking that I could have another 20 years. As I stood there, pondering my future, a man bumped into me and then apologized. "It's my fault," I said, "I shouldn't just be standing here, but I was trying to decide what I am going to do with the rest of my life." I had never seen this man before and I will probably never see him again, but he spent the next ten minutes with me, making suggestions as to what I might do. Oh my, oh my, there can be some delicious moments when they are least expected. I finally ignored my mother's admonitions about not talking to strangers and what fun! Wish I had broken more rules earlier in life. What rules have you broken lately? Consequences?

29. THE EYE OF THE BEHOLDER

The world's a funny place. We each see it in a different way and that's probably why it keeps slipping out of our hands. Just when we think we've got a handle on its operating system, something goes awry, and we no longer have hold of the string.

For instance, when your eyes focus on a glass that's not filled to the top, it's either half empty or half full. How you describe that glass, tells something about you. If you perceive it as half full, you are probably an optimist, but if you say that the glass is half empty, then you're most likely to be more of a pessimist.

Of course that's not written in stone, but those persons who generally are of a more hopeful bent, regard the world and its contents thereof, in a more favorable way. If, like Chicken Little, you are plagued with such worries as "the sky is falling," you may often regard events as tending towards a somewhat, or even complete, catastrophic end.

As I have decided to grow older disgracefully, I have also decided to remove toxins from my life, both things as well as people. For instance, I will no longer dine with those people who, despite having more time on their hands than they could ever use up, complain about the slowness of the wait staff right from the moment they sit down. Dining is supposed to be a pleasurable experience, whereas going to the doctor is not, so if these same people want to complain about waiting at the doctor's office, I will understand, although if they brought along something to read, they wouldn't be so bored and cantankerous.

The longer you live, the more baggage you have in your life, and at times, it takes a conscious effort to look at your world through rose colored glasses - definitely the preferred shade. You can choose to be optimistic about your life or you can be pessimistic. Like the glass, which I mentioned at the beginning of this treatise on the preferred state of mind, you can look back on your life and think of the many wonderful things that you have accomplished and that have filled your life to the brim. Or, you can look back at your life and bemoan the many things you did not accomplish and oh, woe is me. The glass container of your life can be almost full or it can be mostly empty. Your choice. Your point of view is yours alone. Think about it. Which fascinates more, a tale of sorrow or a tale of joy? Me, I'll take the anti-toxin any time.

30. TOO LATE SMART?

If you're willing to learn and you keep on learning, it's not too late to get smart.

In the past months, I have learned how to stop urinary tract infections dead in their tracks, (little pun, there) and how to prevent them altogether. I've learned what to use to restore your nails to their former hardness after removing artificial nails. I've also decided to reveal my secret pill that when taken along with antibiotics, prevents or at least reduces the severity of yeast infections. As for those ugly, discolored toenails, there's an old fashioned remedy that, when placed under nail tips, performs magic. If you're interested, you'll have to contact me because I'm not about to give free advertising space to some major companies. At least, not until they don't charge me for their products. What are those products? I'll tell you, but I won't mention any names on my website until yada, yada, yada.....

There is something else I have known for several years, and the use of these products does make a difference, because friends are always commenting on my youthful skin. No miracles and no chemicals - just some over the counter stuff that really does the trick. I don't own stock in these companies (damn) but I'll pass their names along to you if you contact me.

You know, it's funny, but the other day over lunch, a bunch of us grande dames were discussing what and how we have learned over the years. For example, recipes. Some of the best recipes we have found were in those little PTA books put out by mothers who were members. You know the kind of books, loved by their families and often passed down through generations. Got any of those? I have a swell one for meatballs. Contact me and maybe we can exchange.

By the way, that's not all we have learned. Growing older disgracefully is not for the meek and faint hearted. If you're going to bend the rules you've got to have backbone and at least a soupcon of brashness. Like many of my peers, I watch my pennies and my nickels ad nauseam, and when I reach the cashier's desk at the front, I take my time checking on the" buy one get one free" stuff and any specials at all. And you know mistakes get made. When the register scans the product, there can be errors and the cashiers are sometimes not apprised of changes. Of course, checking out requires time, and waiting customers sometimes get impatient and a tad nasty. I used to get frazzled and try to rush things along but now, I look over my shoulder at the mad mob and sweetly say that I have enough money to buy the sale items, but if anyone is in a hurry and wants to give me the difference in price, I'll gladly pay and leave. No offers yet, but you never know and it does get quieter. How do you deal with the madding crowd?

There used to be a feeling of shame at not having enough money, but with today's new economy, it's politically correct to be poor. In all my years, I was never really in, in fact at times I was so far out, that I was actually in, but today I'm in, really in. Living long and growing older. I knew there was an advantage somewhere, but I was having trouble finding it. Not anymore. I'm with the trendsetters at last. How about you? Are you in or are you out?

31. WHY IS IT SO HARD TO BE KIND?

I'm sure I've said this before but please forgive me. I am growing older disgracefully and sometimes I probably sound like a broken record. Don't give me that look. You know what I mean by the word record. You didn't emerge from the womb with a DVD in your hand, not if we're the same generation.

At any rate, I've been racking my brain, trying to fathom why we have so much difficulty, when it comes to being kind to one another. Is it part of our nature to be mean and uncaring? No, no - well maybe when we were kids, because children can certainly be cruel to one another but then, as we become socialized, we are influenced by parents and teachers and maybe even our peers. As we grow and leave our early state of fragility, we develop an armor that protects us from the slings and arrows - hopefully- and why be nasty when you can be nice, becomes a part of our thinking.

It seems to me, nastiness emerges when our lives begin to change. Not necessarily a purposeful trait, but rather a sort of my life is becoming a bumpy road so why should you have a smoother path than I, sort of thing. The problem - as I see it - is that as we age, we gradually return to that very early stage of fragility and increased awareness of self. We forget that little things, to be totally corny, mean a lot. I will never forget, on the very first day after moving into my senior complex, there was a big party, and as I walked alone, trying to find an available seat, a wonderful couple stopped me and asked me to join them. That's kindness. Don't you agree?

By the way, if you feel offended when you read this, could you just stop reading and walk away. In my world, we don't all come from the same place and sometimes we need to agree to disagree. Expressing dissimilar points of view needn't lead to conflict, concord best achieved if everyone gets to have his or her say. So speak up and listen up. I think that's better than a muzzle or tearing down a poster or a flyer.

Maybe kindness is just walking momentarily in someone else's shoes, and that is difficult because at birth we have a strong sense of I, and then as we acquire spouses and children and friends, we develop a sense of you. Then as we age, we apparently return to the sense of I, because just maintaining oneself becomes more and more difficult. What a pity that is, because often, turning our focus elsewhere, relieves that internal pressure that we feel.

So that makes it simple to be kind, doesn't it? Well, really, if my being kind to you benefits me, that's a no brainer. We'll kill each other with kindness. Just joking. Maybe a little smother now and then. Okay?

32. WHEE! ARE FAMILY

Family. Not something you want to think about before taking your blood pressure, because it's a word often charged with emotion.

Maybe you're one of the exceptional ones and you come from a family like the Waltons - remember John Boy - where never is heard a discouraging word and - well, you get my drift.

But don't count on it. Families are composed of people, and one of the big factors about people, is their unpredictability. For instance, if you're growing older disgracefully and you're in a rule breaking state of mind, now is a good time to throw out the old and bring in the new.

Take a commonly held belief. If your children "turn out" well it's to your credit, and if they're considered a bunch of losers, well, that's your fault, of course. After all you raised them. Not necessarily true. Unless you kept them tied up in the root cellar until they were 18, they've probably been influenced more by their peers than by you.

Family is a comfort to have around when you're growing up. Not just for making your lunch and taking you shopping, but for those moments when you think the world has forgotten or abandoned you, and you need someone who accepts you as you are - most of the time, anyway.

Know something funny? Family is a comfort to have when you've grown old. You might not need anyone to make your lunch but it's possible that you need someone to take you to the supermarket or to the doctor, and you need someone who understands that the difference between 50 and 80 is more than just 30 years.

You need someone who doesn't think that no one has ever carried a burden such as theirs. Yes, they still have children, probably grown, but requiring their ministrations, and now they are torn by responsibility for aging parents. That's not new, the aging parents bit, you had that too. It's part of the mosaic, handed down from generation to generation, only some generations seem to bend while others appear to break.

If you're waiting for a magical solution, I don't have it. Maybe if I had been clever enough to come up with Face book or even a way to allow elderly persons to buy their medications, along with an occasional lobster or sirloin steak, maybe I would be the one to solve all family problems. What I do believe, is that those of us who were enlightened enough to accept our families as they were, may still be able to recapture that same sense of enlightenment and accept our families as they are today. Maybe. Maybe the jury is still out? But maybe not.

33. THEY HAVE THEIR HANDS IN YOUR POCKETS

Hey there! We're not going to let you do it. We may be old but one thing we have learned. In union there is strength, and we're going to join our hands and keep your hands out of our pockets.

We're not going to pay for the stupid wars that take the lives of our vital young people. My father used to say that we should send the old people to war. They would look at each other, put down their guns, take out a deck of cards and winner takes all. All except lives and what else is really important and irreplaceable?

Social Security was put in place a long time ago and it has worked incredibly well. And would continue to do so until the elected officials that we put in place, decide that we give too much to the people in this country. Handouts, they call them, but it's not a handout when you give people back the money that the government set aside from their wages, so that they can have something to sustain them in their old age.

    Why do the people need this money, anyway? Why didn't they put their money away for their retirement, instead of splurging on housing and food and clothing for their kids and money for college? They should have earned more money like the wealthy 1% of people in this country. Granted, not everyone can inherit their wealth but everyone can work harder. After all this is America and all men are created equal and if you dispute that, you're a communist or a socialist or maybe just an old curmudgeon and that's equally bad.

    Call me irascible or even irresistible, but don't pay for your damn wars by stealing from our Social Security or Medicare. If we'd known you guys were going to have such good personal medical coverage and pensions, we would have junked all the fuss about the Electoral College and concentrated our efforts on paring down your benefits. We make being a member of congress too appealing. It should be a privilege to serve your country and you should not need any further rewards. If you keep hammering away at our social security and Medicare, we're going to chip away at your perks and then who'll be sorry now?

And fellow grouches, don't let this election slip through your fingers. Find out who's running and what their stance has been on social security and Medicare in the past. Right now they're all for us oldies, but give them our votes and they'll call our entitlements handouts, and reduce us to the status of beggars. Keep an eye on these politicians. They have elevated taking other people's money, to high art. Vote early and often - whatever it takes.

34. SILK PURSE OR SOW'S EAR?

Please, no more dancing in the rain, and take your bowl of cherries and stick that where the rain is, too. All this sugar is not good for our aging arteries and it's about time we called what it is, what it is. That's the glory of growing older disgracefully. You can make a mountain out of a mole hill or insist that a pile of dung will not smell any sweeter because you change its name. All these little ditties about how you get up in the morning and do a little jig to greet the day. Heck, you're happy if you can move your aching back to the sink and brush your teeth. If you still call the time of aging the golden years, your powers of perception have tarnished along with lots of other stuff.

Sure, we say that this is the time to do what you

want, but the issue is not what you want, but rather of what you are capable. The sun is so bright and you're ready to climb a mountain, but first you have to climb down the steps. There's that little thing. Why are all these paeans to the glories of life, written by bright eyed and bushy tailed youngsters? Because they have control of all of their moving parts, both internal and external, and they haven't yet experienced rust.

I'm the eternal optimist, but my years have changed me into the unwavering realist. This is not the best of all times, although I won't let it degenerate into the worst of all times. I just insist that it is what it is and I refuse to dwell in an ivory tower. Was life more romantic when there were more wrinkles in my clothes than on my face? Yeah, sure, but romance has evolved into a good night's sleep and fewer visits to the toilet during the night. And speaking of visits, let's throw in fewer visits to my doctor.

As someone where I live, answered, when a friend told her that she always looks as though she's going to a party, "When I wake up every day and feel good and see the sun, I am going to a party." Good way to think, as long as you don't plan to dance in the rain. Staying upright on a slippery street is enough of a challenge. Isn't it? 'Tis. 'Tis.

35. LOVE IN THE AFTERNOON

When we smile, our faces may crinkle up with wrinkles, and there are many silver threads among the gold or red or brown, but that doesn't mean that we don't still tear up when we watch some lovely romance on screen, and think of how nice it would be if we could throw away our canes and dance.

Of course if we did have a dalliance, it would have to be in the afternoon, because so many of us don't like to drive after it gets dark, and that goes for both the guys and dolls. A nice stroll on the beach would be romantic, although we might have to compromise for a stroll near the beach, because our walkers do have a tendency to get bogged down in the sand.

For me, just playing some tender music, sitting

on my porch watching cars go by, seeing the leaves rustle on the big tree outside my screen - well that just pushes my remember romance button, and if I close my eyes, I travel back in time. You know that expression about letting your fingers do the walking. In my case, my mind does the walking and I'm back somewhere far away and I feel kind of melty - you remember that feeling - and you all of a sudden realize that maybe something is missing.

I have lots of friends (gal pals) and there's always something to do to keep yourself occupied but sometimes, when I'm alone in my apartment at night - for instance, having watched a DVD like the one I watched last night about Queen Victoria and her consort, Prince Albert - and how deeply they were in love (After he died, she had his clothes laid out for him every day until the day she died). That's deep alright, and I did get a bit teary, and for a moment I thought about the excitement of falling in love. Ahh - Then I thought about blood pressure and heart stress and the pain of unrequited love. Too much pain if you're dealing with arthritis and general joint pain. Besides, as you grow older disgracefully, you tend to have some sleep problems and you don't want "does he or she love me, or love me not?" added to the other burning questions which tend to pop up in the middle of the night. Still, am I missing something? Am I?

Evelyn Marder Levin

Play it again, Sam. Please do.

36. WELCOME TO HAPPY HOUR

I'm told that where they live, many people attend a monthly or even weekly happy hour. Does that mean that every 7 or 3o days they can expect to feel joy?? So what do they feel the rest of the time? Goofy, if they ask silly questions like this. But seriously, I do wonder sometimes how this period of forced merriment, originally rising out of a bottle, came into being.

A little research uncovered the origin of happy hour as being related to prohibition in the United Sates (the Volstead Act), when people would get together before dinner to drink the forbidden fruit of the vine. Of course, alcohol consumption has been legal for many years but the fact that it was forbidden at one time, has added a certain cachet.

Take pot, for instance, I don't, but the governor of my former state, would like to legalize it, and then we could have a stoned hour as well. For many reasons, I don't think that will catch on as has the happy hour. The name, for instance. We who are growing older disgracefully, see happiness as a state of great achievement. We want our children and grandchildren to achieve that state, but as for being stoned - I don't think so.

However, I would like to see the name, happy hour, changed perhaps to the happy period, lasting longer and occurring more frequently. No, I'm not some sort of lush, wanting to add to our alcohol consumption. On the contrary, like so many of my vintage (little pun there) some drink and some don't. It's not important. What is important is adding merriment, happiness, and or joy to our lives on a regular basis.

To be honest, I want all of our hours to be happy. Why do we seem to have so much down time in proportion to the time which can be categorized as up? Well, maybe I'm being a bit greedy. How about more clumps of happy seconds, sprinkled hither and yon throughout the day? When you least expect it? A surprise, so to speak. I'm all for surprises. Good ones, of course, although if you're like me and believe that anticipation is all, then surprises are not always so fun.

That sentence needed a modifier, but I'm learning to be cool like my offspring. I can text, I'm on Face book, I twitter. Hours of happiness will soon be mine, as will large bills for my texting, but I will drown my cares at happy hour - the original - and happy days, as well.

37. DAY LIFE SAVINGS TIME

    Two older women meet in the elevator. "What's new?" asks one. The second woman says, "I have good news and bad news." "What's the good news?" "Today is my birthday." "Congratulations, and what's the bad news?" "Today is my birthday."

    Birthdays are usually pleasurable, and as you age, each additional one is a way of marking another year of life. Yes, there comes a time when you no longer believe you're going to live forever and in the senior complex in which I live, some people say their good nights, adding, "See you in the morning - I hope." When you're young, the thought of not being here forever is too difficult to contemplate, but part of growing older disgracefully is telling yourself that you've had a good run and all good things end sometime.

However, I couldn't help thinking, on my recent birthday, that it would pretty neat if we could turn back the clock - not permanently- just on occasion - calling it day life savings time. There's no point in really going back, because without the experience and wisdom that, hopefully you have acquired, you would just make the same decisions you had made before. No, what I have in mind is something more delicious, an actual reliving of some wonderful moment or moments that took place in your life, and that you would enjoy reliving. For me, it was back to a time when I was assistant director of Career Planning at a college, and because I was an "alum" of that college, the students asked me to give their class day speech. I had spoken in front of small groups, but this was to be in front of parents, faculty and students. I remember telling the students that someday one of them might be the President of the United States and that I was sure, that whoever she was, she would do an outstanding job. I can still almost hear the cheers and applause when I said that.

Afterwards, what I remember most vividly, was when a member of the faculty came up to me and said that he had heard more speeches than he had hairs on his head, (no, he wasn't bald) and he didn't think that he would ever hear anything new, but my speech had proven him wrong. Of course, going back would mean reliving the shaking of my knees, and the nervous preparation that preceded my standing in front of what seemed like a huge crowd of people, but I felt great joy and a sense of accomplishment. Not so many of those moments nowadays, but the same feelings when they occur. Wish I had more of them. How about you?

38. THE BODY HAS A HEAD

Hey, we knew that. Guess that growing older disgracefully is sometimes just growing older in terms of our brain and its capabilities. A little dementia going on there, with the need to point out that the body has a head. It also has two arms and two legs and lots of other quite obvious stuff.

But that's not what I meant, what I meant is that the body has a mind and the mind directs the body and how it functions. Let's take some examples. For instance, your blood pressure. We all have certain stressors and when we can't contain them, our blood pressure starts to soar. You know how it is when you get into that shoulda, coulda, woulda kind of stuff. You tense up, and when you're upset, your adrenal glands release adrenaline into your body, affecting your heart beat and your blood vessels and ultimately affecting your blood pressure. Lack of sleep affects your blood pressure. The sleep process helps your heart to slow down and your entire body to relax. Deep breathing is another way of relaxing your body, especially the type of breaths that involve your diaphragm and enable you to breathe as deeply as possible.

We have learned that certain exercises can lower your blood pressure. Some people have found meditation to be a way of releasing stressors from the mind and thereby from the body. The mind body connection affects all areas of the body, from headaches to stomach aches to weakening of our immune system. People spend a great deal of time and concern regarding what they eat, which, of course, is important, but we should also be giving thought to what is eating us.

I don't usually recommend a particular book, but I found a recently published book at my library and it might be called a primer for dealing with elevated blood pressure. It's title is "Bringing Down High Blood Pressure" and the authors are Chad Rhoden, M.D., Ph.D. with Sarah Wiley Schein, M.S., R.D., L.D.N.. It's simply written so that you don't need a medical degree to understand it, and it's presented chapter by chapter, outlining the steps you can take to reduce your blood pressure. Also, for those of us who have been inundated with cholesterol figures to the exclusion of other important body numbers, there's an explanation as to why blood pressure is so important and how we can learn to take charge.

Let's keep in mind that growing older disgracefully is being in control of our bodies whenever we can. Maybe we can't still run a marathon, but many of us can still run rings around those who have fewer rings around their trunks.

39. VALENTINE'S DAY – WHAT'S LOVE GOT TO DO WITH IT?

When I was in grade school, Valentine's Day became a contest to see who would get the greatest number of cards from classmates, regardless of sexual orientation. Love put aside, it was strictly a numbers game, and contingent on the quantity and awareness of one's friends, at the end of the day, you could have won or lost. Love had nothing to do with it and that kind of simplified things. Take love out of the equation and lots of things get simpler, but that's cynical old me speaking and not some starry eyed youngster.

Over the years, Valentine's Day came and went as did the cards, flowers and gifts, as our levels of sophistication grew, along with the importance of love or caring in some of its various guises, pertaining to The Day. When our offspring were little, cards were exchanged all around and big red boxes of chocolate candies for mommy became de rigueur. The cards were mushy and sentimental and probably unappreciated, because who knew we were going through a phase that was most certainly not going to last forever? Who knew that the ocean would become a river and then a stream and trickle on down to not much at all? Who knew? Who knew?

Not I, said the little red hen, remembering that I used to send cards to my sons well into manhood (theirs, not mine). Cards also went to their peripherals - spouses, kids etc.. It was fun to buy them, almost as much fun as to receive them. And then the music stopped. No spouses, no lovers, no boyfriends, no cards. We entered the territory of sporadic. You know where that is - somewhere between occasionally, infrequently and never.

Did I initiate the crossover? Maybe. I don't remember. But then, since I've joined we who are growing older disgracefully, I don't remember lots of things. Anyway, it's not really of vital importance. What has occurred to me is how we seem to go full circle in life.

Valentine's Day came and went and the number

of cards etc. had little to do with caring and love, it was more a contest of numbers. Now here we are back to the numbers. I received one card. Should we revive the old traditions? Texting and emails are for words. Envelopes are for enclosures. Some of us have gone from empty nests to empty envelopes. Beyond our control, and love has nothing to do with it? Does it? Does it? I think not.

40. IF YOU WERE THE ONLY BOY

... in the world and I....well, you know how that goes. Takes me all the way back to high school when a girl couldn't have a friend who was a boy, or a boy couldn't have a friend who was a girl. No, they had to be boyfriend/girlfriend with all the baggage that goes with such a relationship. It wasn't until you were grown up, that you began to realize that having a friendship - no strings attached - with a member of the opposite sex could be quite rewarding in ways that you didn't expect. For instance, you learned how men often think differently than women, a fact which became quite helpful in your business dealings, as well as in your search for a mate. Of course, to be perfectly honest, dealings with the opposite sex provides a little harmless titillation, or so it is said.

Another wonderful discovery was how utilitarian it is to have someone who could help with a tight jar lid, or could sew on a button that stayed put. So the years passed, and you had many friends, and when you didn't feel like dishing with the girls, you could have a spirited discussion about whose team was going to lead the field. I don't wish to sound sexist, but gals have dishing down to a fine art. Most often, though, as the years pile on, the guys seem to be able to dish almost as well, and with equal enthusiasm.

And so things just went along until you began to grow older disgracefully, and part of that journey included a return trip to adolescence - obviously - because it was observed that your aging friends could no longer be just friends, they had to be boyfriends / girlfriends. Not a rule, of course, but prevalent enough to merit notice. Why oh why is that so?

In my senior community, apparently as well as in many others, the search for exclusivity in a companion - often initiated by the females, since they are in the majority- frequently leads to what seemingly, at times, is a battleground. There are emanations of he's mine - hands off - and a simple conversation is viewed with suspicion. Can't we all just be friends and not become an "item" because we dine at the same table? I guess not. Thus be it ever and creaking bones and all, the chase is on. More of a sock hop than a chase, but it does go on. And on.

41. STAND YOUR GROUND........OH, DO SIT DOWN

    Since that rule has been dredged out, everyone wants to get even, and instant retribution has replaced even the smallest instant of reflection. The horrendous movie theatre incident, where a man lost his life for texting, was doubly chilling in light of the airlines' possible lifting of its ban on use of cell phones, when aloft. Whoo -eeee! Don't like having to listen to that conversation and the one next to you is no better? Well it's no bang bang, because guns are prohibited on board (unless you're a law enforcement officer - hmm??) but I think there's a much more serious issue at stake.

    We're a very crowded country, as you're well

aware, if you've ever lived in a big city, and we seem to be getting more obsessive about our space. But that seems to be true everywhere, even where there's lots more space around us. Sitting in an office, waiting to be served in a cafe, trying to pass the time by reading our books. Quite impossible. There are people all around us, talking, laughing, just generally impacting on our trains of thought. Most annoying, but what to do? Nothing! There is nothing to do except maybe to become more expert at concentrating on the subject at hand, or close our eyes and get a few winks. Don't worry - you'll hear your name when it's called.

The senior complex in which I live, despite its many good features, abounds in complaints. The dining room is too noisy, people's voices are too loud and I'm told the reason for this is that many people are hearing impaired and hearing aids are often not aids at all. People wear too much scent or not enough. The elevators are crowded or too few and yet I believe the average wait never exceeds three minutes. Also, the people who are waiting are all retired and have more time than probably the years left to spend it.

So what is it we want, anyway? Is it just we who are growing older disgracefully who are struggling with issues of patience and tolerance, or is the whole world metaphorically prepared to stand its ground, come what may? Maybe we need a little old fashioned duel challenging? Ah, there's an idea and if we can replace bullets with cream puffs, I'm ready to stand at fifty paces. Right now.

42. DREAM, WHEN YOU'RE FEELING BLUE

Well your dreams belong to you, don't they? You and someone else and not always by invitation. Sometimes by intrusion. Sometimes by inclusion. Sometimes you think you're in a room full of strangers and then the person you've been waiting for comes in, and you're suffused with joy. The room was empty and now it's full. But wait, it's full all right but there's no joy. Where is the one we have been waiting for all our lives?

Please no excuses. I don't want to fight with you. I remember when you were just a baby and everything you did was pure happiness. We who are growing older disgracefully look back at our dreams and see only bliss. Do we dream selectively, seeing only what we allow to remain and sending everything else to the recycling bin?

Wouldn't it be nice to dream whenever you were in the mood, just by lying down and closing your eyes and being able to stop your dreams via the alarm clock, or just by sheer will power, or by making the train the setting of your dreams, and reaching the stop where you get off?

See, since my dreams belong to me there's no "he said, she said," just a return to never, never land and the way I wanted it to be. Or maybe it really was that way and dreamland was just an affirmation.

Anyway, I have been having some seriously wacky dreams and I assume it has plenty to do with what has been going on in my life. I wish I could push the rewind button and go back to where I think I could change my life, though I know it's not possible. I want to say "I love you, I love you, you're perfect", to everyone who crosses the threshold of my dreams. Impossible, so maybe I'll just say more, "you're perfects", to those who cross the threshold of my conscious. Maybe. Are you perfect? Maybe one of us is. Maybe none of us is. So dream.

43. BOOTS ARE MADE FOR WALKING

Now, PETA, don't get your fur balls in an uproar. My boots were faux-fur lined - no polyesters were destroyed to make them - although in my earlier, less enlightened days, I did own some unfaux-fur garments, but even then I never had much use for PETA. I believe that every person should answer to the conscience that was installed at the time of construction, and we should not rely on a universal conscience for our own straight and narrow. That said, let's go marching on to my faux fur lined boots.

As with many persons who were not born in the South, we northerners regard Florida as the land of perpetual warmth and the skies are not cloudy all day, although there is more than a bit of rain at times. Therefore, before heading south, I divested myself of almost all of my cold weather garments, keeping a few, because my daughter in law warned me that the skies might not be cloudy, but they were also not always sunny and baby, sometimes it was COLD outside. I kept my boots because when you've been brought up with the imminence of ice and snow, it always hovers in the back of your mind, come winter. And unlike mowing the lawn, you can't postpone shoveling snow until you're in the mood. Which in my case was never, but that's a whole different tale.

Less than two weeks before Xmas and the temperature drops to 50 degrees. In NY I would put on a jacket, but in Florida, out come the ski jackets, the caps and the gloves. The gleeful TV anchor predicts even cooler temperatures and at night it has dropped to below 40 degrees. My plants did not bring any winter tarps with them, so this afternoon, with a prediction of a hard frost tonight and temperatures perhaps in the thirties, I drag in all my plants, which seem heavier the second time around. Good for my muscles, I grunt to myself, with a chorus of what doesn't kill you makes you stronger.

I don't care. Tomorrow I will wear my faux fur lined boots, boots which I wear in NYC when the snow has fallen and the ice has formed, but that's never going to happen here. I don't care if the eyebrows get raised, because that's part and parcel of growing older disgracefully. I will know I'm being true to myself and isn't that what it's all about? Or maybe they're just jealous.

44. THE WIZARD OF OZ

In the complex where I live, from 3PM to 4PM, Monday through Friday, many of us are fixated on our television sets, listening for words of wisdom from a man the networks call Dr. Oz. I refer to him as the wizard of Oz because the words he sends our way every afternoon are often miraculous to some of us.

Thanks to him, I have found a way to lower my cholesterol so that I may soon drop my cholesterol lowering medication, according to my doctor. My neighbor has lowered her blood pressure, and another friend has dropped a few pounds. Although his studio audience is, on average, considerably younger than the residents where I live, we all have a similar goal - living longer while at the same time living healthier.

When I see his studio audience, who appear to be generally - with some exceptions - amply nourished, although not necessarily well nourished, I wonder how they are going to age. Habits that we form in our early years seem to stay with us as we age, despite efforts to change them. As a long time chocoholic, I understand food addictions very well. Ice cream is another food that I find difficult to resist, especially if it consists of lots of chocolate and nuts.

As I have previously stated, growing older disgracefully means pleasing yourself without being overly concerned with what others think of you. I still believe that, but I also believe that you have to be honest with yourself. If you can say that you really don't give a darn about being overweight, that those love handles you have grown make you feel sexy, that having moved up a size or two when you go shopping, is meaningless - it's only a number- then go for it. Of course, you should be factoring in the side issues, other than aesthetics, that accompany weight gain. For instance, increased risk of diabetes, stress on your body that added weight brings, such as your joints, oh, and that organ called a heart.

Exercise is good, but exercising your will power at the grocery store is good, too. If it's not on your shelves or the menu, you can't eat it, unless, like a compulsive eater I once knew, you get so desperate you send yourself a candy gram. No, that was not me - I have my limits - and I hope I didn't give you any ideas.

45. TO RESOLVE OR NOT TO RESOLVE

As the new year begins, there is always a matter requiring our full attention. Do we make New Year's resolutions or do we not? On the positive side, resolutions provide an official mark- hooray, the New year is here and we can start all over - leaving behind that maybe not so hot old year. Yes, we can forget those broken resolutions. They weren't what we really wanted, anyway. Who actually wanted to lose 10 lbs and exercise at least 5 times a week? Not I, said the little red hen, laughing at the silliness of what we had resolved.

However, on the negative side, resolutions have a certain je ne sais quoi quality, causing them to vanish, sometimes as early as the second week of the month of January. The problem is, that as we grow older disgracefully, we become enlightened as to the futility of changing our slothful ways, especially by making some promises to ourselves that we have no intention of keeping. Or maybe, initially, we do intend to keep them, but on second thoughts, we realized that they were unsuitable to our life styles.

The fault, as I see it, is not in the act of making resolutions, the fault lies in the type of resolutions we make. Remember, we have reached a point in our lives when we do not want to deceive ourselves, and we should employ complete honesty in choosing resolutions that we may possibly keep. I have given a great deal of thought to this, and based on the resolutions which I have made, over the past several years, and which I have never broken, I offer several suggestions.

My first resolution is this: I will never - despite any sort of provocation- chase lions in the street. Unbroken. My second resolution, again, despite any opportunities which may arise: I will never bring an elephant to live with me, into my home. Unbroken.

Now, before you disparage the importance of my resolutions, let me point out how valuable they are. I eliminate any negativity which may arise, immediately tainting a new year with the feeling that I have failed at something, right from the start. No, based on my kept resolutions, I can predict that the coming year will be a success.

I invite you to try out my resolutions this year, and I predict you will experience a similar success. Go ahead, just try them, and please let me know if they have worked out as well for you, as they have for me.

Here's to a wonderful New Year! I promise. You will see.

46. I KNOW HOW YOU FEEL .... DO YOUOOOOO?

Well really? Do You? When I was born I was connected to my Mom by means of an umbilical cord, not a USB cord and maybe that's the first reason that you have no idea how I feel. My old car squeaks its way into my car port parking space, and the adjacent new car eases in like a thief in the night with nary a sound. No aches and pains - not yet - but its day will come and then it can make all the noises it wants. My car and I, we've put in the time. We know how we feel but you don't know until you know, so please, let me be old in peace.

Where I live, no one is old; we're all mature, but we have grab bars in the shower, old lady/man toilet seats in the bathroom and emergency cords near the bed, not as you might have thought, for room service, but just emergency services for you. This is the first place I have lived, where sirens in the night do not mean a police raid for those noisy party givers upstairs, just a trip to the local hospital and no party.

I finally got the hang of email. I like it as much as anyone who knows the power of the written word and has exercised it to advantage in the past. I've even been able to ignore a lack of confidentiality, particularly as I'm not a Governor or any such holder of high government office, but I am defeated by Face book. I don't understand how to send a private message or maybe you're not supposed to. I call it faceless book because it seems to me one picture or one phrase fits all. No, I don't know how you feel. I don't text because I never learned to type. In my day, girls who could type became secretaries. So I didn't.

I struggle to be with it, and that means a lot of tough work at the computer. I also spend a lot of time learning how to use the digital camera and how to upload the pictures that I take. I had so many nice cameras and a dark room that went obsolete, as will I, and so will you. No, you don't know how I feel, but you will, and you'll say that old so and so, she could have given us a clue. Then at last you'll really know how I feel. Lucky, lucky you, you'll feel it, too.

47. DELAYED GRATIFICATION

Delay? Not in my brain or vocabulary. If I wanted it, I would get it because I could. If something was advertised and it looked appealing, I would pick up the phone or my mouse and soon it was on its way. Oh of course, it had to be affordable, but that's a very flexible word and open to much interpretation. One man or woman's affordable, is someone else's splurge and somehow, when the regularity of hefty paychecks had become a given, frugality took a back seat. But now it has become the driver and sits up front, where it belongs.

The funny thing is, it hasn't much impacted my life. Does that speak to a change in my thought processes or just to the change in my disposable income? Had I been buying into the belief that things would improve my life and perhaps even make me more satisfied? For many people, shopping, or acquiring, is a goal, an occupation, a form of entertainment. Is it all of those things because we can afford it to be, or would we make it affordable, no matter what, because it is so important to our lives and fills a desire?

At the moment of desire, are we having more fun than budgeting and planning, which involves making sacrifices. Or do we? It's a conundrum - that's the kind of word that I use when I'm truly - this is actually a good place for the past tense of a 4 letter word but in deference to those who grow older gracefully I will abstain - Use whatever word you will, but it is puzzling and it is always difficult for us to define ourselves.

A lot of words, as the old Bard would have said, words signifying nothing and perhaps that is true, but as I grow older, I need to question my values, and in so doing, find a way to value my life. Postponing gratification has brought a feeling of achievement into my life. I can be happy with what I have and I need less.

I think I know where I am. One night, a group of residents where I live, discussed what plans they would make if they won the Lotto. Money for children, travel, college tuition - all commendable choices, but I had decided a while back - I would take the bulk of my money and set up a foundation to help old persons in need. I'm not homeless and I have enough to eat, but old age is tough, and unless you have a working crystal ball- well, you know about the best laid plans.

Delay? In my vocabulary, only not things, but days, hours, moments. I wake up and the day is mine and my Daisy is whining for her breakfast. What a wonderful sound! Oh, and the rent is paid. We'll work out everything else.

48. HAPPY HOLIDAY, ALL RIGHT, ALREADY

"Have a wonderful Thanksgiving. Do you have any special plans?"

"Getting together with your family?" "Who's making the dinner?"

We meet one another and we assume that this widely celebrated holiday is truly a widely celebrated holiday. Like many holidays, family is the operant word and sometimes we forget that having a family is not always a given, and that at times, not having a family may be a blessing. I know, there are those who say - with a tone of disparagement- that you've never met my family, but because we're growing older disgracefully, we have somehow learned to forgive and accept.

One of the many myths about the first

thanksgiving is that the hunters returned after massacring Indians and celebrated their victory at a dinner of thanks. Of course the story has evolved, and whatever its origins, Thanksgiving has become a ritual involving too much food and too much stuffing and I don't mean only the turkey.

This is not a time for guilt over diets broken. This is a time of plenty, too much plenty, if we can express ourselves in such an ungrammatical way. If, as many claim, food is love, then this is the time that we express our love in each course that comes to the table. In every luscious bite of corn bread and every piece of home baked pie.

Thanksgiving seemingly marks the start of the holiday season, the winter madness that begins with shopping until everyone on our voluminous lists has been gifted. Ah, but I have decided that this year is going to be different. Like so many seniors, to whom the phrase "cost of living" has become a political baseball, with the seniors striking out, I have to consult an actuary to estimate how many more years I can afford to live, and what I need to cut back on if, heaven forbid, he gives me more years than I have budgeted for.

I have devised a tier system of gift-giving. The absolute musts, the maybes and the ones who find me as much of a chore as I find them. How can I tactfully inform my dear ones that I don't need any more "things". I haven't figured out a system of taking things when I go, so would it be all right if I had a T shirt printed up with "cash is king" across the front. Too subtle? We could do the back with "No amount too small", as well.

49. IT'S AIRPORT SCAN, NOT SCAM

I'm on the scan bandwagon. Ever since I read about the young man who managed to get on a plane with a bomb in his underpants, I've been convinced that we should let it all hang out. I don't care. I say that it's better to be red than dead, and besides, have you observed your fellow passengers lately? It's like going to the beach. You may feel self-conscious in your swim suit until you look around at the yards of flesh being uncovered, and with seeming unselfconsciousness, in many cases.

So what's the big deal, anyway? Not being so touchy feely as many, I would much prefer a little undercover viewing, to being patted down in various places. There are no dangerous rays resulting from a body scan, unless you are actually hiding an explosive device in your intimate garments and then, of course, there will be consequences. Someone suggested that the body scanners should have a mechanism built into them, so that when they are in use and encounter an explosive device such as a bomb, they set off a mini explosion, with just enough force to make the privates of the person being scanned, become public. I have no idea about the logistics of such a step, since even setting off fireworks makes me nervous, but there must be people out there, who are expert in the art of blowing things up.

I do believe, since I am committed to growing older disgracefully, that the safest way to grow older, even as an infrequent flyer, is to be vigilant, since there are those who are apparently committed to keeping many Americans from growing older at all. We can put our heads in the sand and say that we take terrorism too seriously, but the victims of terrorism (if they were still here) would dispute that statement.

In this country, we take people's lives as a serious issue. We protect lives whenever we can, and we never consider a human body as part of an explosive device. People are not bombs and we do not employ them as such to win a war. We do not condone human sacrifice as a guarantee for eternal

Paradise. Actually, we offer prayers and we make promises which we try to keep, but guarantees - that would be a scam and not a scan, and like we told you, we're just talking about scans at the airport. How does all of this grab you?

50. REACH OUT AND TOUCH SOMEONE

These words have been going through my mind since the day after Thanksgiving. Black Friday, it is called, but for me the meaning was far from that of the retail community, referring to Christmas sales.

In the complex where I live, a woman took her life by jumping eight stories to her death. I didn't really know this woman or the circumstances of her life, but I have had several somewhat sleepless nights, trying to understand how it is possible for a human being to forfeit what seems to me the most wonderful gift of all - the gift of life.

Those of us who live in this community have by and large, lived through at least seven or eight decades of life and some even nine. Recalling my own life and those of others I have known, I have learned that life isn't a given. Still births, accidents, diseases, all seeming opponents of being alive and staying alive, keep us vigilant, and sadden us at times, but at other times we are filled with gratitude.

Philosophers have pondered the nature of life, trying to explain its origins, and men of medicine search for ways to expand and improve the duration, as well as the quality of life. Poets eulogize what they consider the beautiful in life, and you and I question and simultaneously heap praise and condemnation on an amazing force that we don't really understand, but for which we still give thanks.

Yes, living is indeed a slippery slope and there are times, without exception, when each and every one of us needs a hand. Sadly, some of us don't know how to ask, or consider that our asking for help is a sign of weakness, so imbued are we with being stouthearted, and filled with the dogma that every one of us is an island. But of course, we are not.

No man or woman is an island, as postulated by the poet, John Donne, "Any man's death diminishes me, Because I am so involved in mankind, And therefore never send to know for whom the bell tolls; it tolls for thee." If we truly believe that, it is beholden on every one of us to reach out and touch someone. Maybe we didn't always behave in that fashion, but as older citizens who are committed to growing older disgracefully, I am convinced that our time is now. Are you with me? Are you ready to reach out and touch someone? Now?

51. ANIMAL CRACKERS IN MY SOUP

It's time to speak of one of the most important - if not the most important - beings in my life, my dog, Daisy.

Daisy is a 13 year old Yorkshire Terrier, with the soul and spirit of a puppy, who astonishes everyone with her joie de vivre and her adorable face. I'm still struggling with my new digital camera, but with Daisy's help, I should soon be able to upload her picture.

During the 13 years we have been together, we have bonded completely. She has allowed me to sleep in her bed, no great sacrifice on her part, because it is full size, and when that little body snuggles up against me, all is very right with my world.

When we first became acquainted and started

out on our journey together, I promised her that I would respect the fact of her being a dog and there would be no silly clothes and no equally silly tricks. Despite that pledge, she has, on her own, learned to spell the word "treat," less from any great skill on her part and any drilling on mine, and rather more from the word's repeatedly being spelled when I thought I was being clever. So now when I spell, do you want a "t r e a t," she sits at the ready.

She also has learned the meaning of some constantly repeated other words, such as "go back to sleep it's too early" - this at any time in the A.M. before seven, and "go to sleep, it's late" -this at any time after 9 P.M. when she has jumped off the bed. Thus, we are able to converse with one another, although I sometimes have to remind her to knock it off. Still, as I spend much time at the computer, a solitary occupation, it's wonderful to have a constant companion, who gives kisses in return for food.

My big concern vis-a-vis Daisy, is her longevity or lack of. With luck, being of a small breed, she may live another 6 years and perhaps we can go to the happy hunting ground together. Some people regard my feelings as being morbid, but part of growing older disgracefully, is the ability to be grateful for what your past life has been, while facing your future head on. After all, what is quantity time without the accompanying good quality? I believe that how we live is in our hands. How long we live is in a different set of hands. Do you agree? What are your thoughts?

52. OPPOSABLE THUMBS, WHO NEEDS THEM?

Not my Daisy. That's for sure. She couldn't be more perfect, even if she could open the refrigerator door and bring me a large glass of iced coffee to slake my afternoon thirst. Coffee, which, by the way we, who are growing older disgracefully, have just been informed will be of benefit by acting as a stimulus and waker – upper, to those who fall asleep in front of the TV in the afternoon. Although, in my opinion, I believe that better programming would also be a stimulus. However, no one has asked my opinion, so back to Daisy.

She is my 4 legged daughter and our relationship was cemented 13 years ago, when we became family. To dog and other animal lovers, I do not need to explain our familial relationship and to those who consider animals an inferior species, there is no possibility of an explanation. So there we have it. Daisy and I have lived and loved together for more than 13 years. I have sons who have been family for many times the multiple of 13 and they do have opposable thumbs, but they find a visit to me to be fraught with difficulty, so one can only imagine how involved a glass of iced coffee from the refrigerator would be.

Anyway, this morning I took my little Yorkie, named Daisy, to her Veterinary Doctor for her annual checkup. Daisy, who weighs 6lbs, has lost some weight because last year she started to limp and it seemed she was having a problem with her Patella (kneecap) which refused to stay in place but which resumed its rightful place and remained there when she lost I lb. Daisy went on a diet, cut back on her treats, added string beans (hates French cut - loves Italian chunk) and sweet peppers, and goes for a walk, which I kindly take with her every day. Not a totally unselfish act, more one of mutual benefit.

    She passed her physical with flying colors and our doc told us that obesity is a problem with dogs as well as people, and just like humans, it impacts their aging years. If Daisy departs this earth before I, it will be losing a member of the family and without discussion, I know she will feel the same about me and it's more than being about opposable thumbs. As a nature show junkie on Public TV, I have learned that animals have an incredible sense of family and its ties. We are speaking of animals in the wild, who base their actions and emotions on instinct, which in turn is based on love.

Daisy and I understand that, and we don't put too much stock in the thumbs. Sure, I have the thumbs, but she has that warm, furry body which she lets me stroke - the best soporific in the world. If you have an animal in your life, I say thumbs up. Lucky, lucky you.

Coda: As of now, Daisy is not so high on string beans, unless they are frozen and mixed with canned, pure mashed pumpkin. I hate pumpkin! Go figure?

53. PUTTING ON THE DOG

Quite literally, that's exactly what we're doing. We're putting me - Daisy, the dog - on the grrouch.com blog. Why are we doing this? Because my mother (strictly adoptive) decided that after 13 years of bonding, I should also become a spokesperson for our team.

We are both growing older disgracefully, but if you'll pardon a bit of tail wagging and bragging, I think I have a slight edge. I mean my 4 legs seem to function better than her 2 and although a bit of gray has touched my hair, not a single drop of Clairol or L'Oreal has been allowed to modify my beautiful fur coat. Admittedly, having a fur coat in Florida is not necessarily such an advantage, but being able to walk around unclothed, certainly is.

A little bit about me. I'm a Yorkshire Terrier,

weighing in at under 6 lbs, which means I'm quite trim- not by choice, but I can't reach the treats - or much of anything, except the bed, and I sleep a lot. I have many opinions and I'm going to use this as a forum to express them. For starters, humans should be seen and not heard, unless they have something worth saying and how often does that happen? Barks should be used more frequently as warnings than as greetings. A little woof is enough to use to greet an old friend, while an ear shattering bark is ok to warn off a perceived enemy, and since they all seem like enemies, better to be safe than to be sorry, I say.

One thing which we do pretty regularly is walk. I'm a civilized pooch and have learned to use the facilities in the house (a box on the porch) for my personal needs, but sometimes, being with just the one person all the time, life gets a little tedious. So, in the hot season we walk inside and when it cools off, we go out into nature. She thinks we're walking to keep me strong. I think we're doing it for her, but isn't that what love is all about?

Nice thing about getting older disgracefully is that things you used to worry about don't seem important any more. For instance, I used to worry that my bow was on crooked or that some of the other dogs got more treats than me, or that some wore fancy clothes, but I don't even like clothes, so that was kind of silly. I'm not alone very much. My mother stays home with me and when she goes out she gives me the most incredible chicken treats ever----and she never, ever forgets. Since this is my introduction, I'm being very positive, but I'll have some complaints when the occasion rises. I'm not very dogmatic, but I like to speak my mind from time to time, and doggone it, I will!

54. ALL IN THE FAMILY

As I may have mentioned, earlier, I was going to add my opinion to this book, so here I am, Daisy, the canine member of this family, such as it is. I say that, because I was separated from my birth mother and family at a very early age and have, apparently, made a very satisfactory adjustment to my adoptive mother. In fact, I have no regrets. I would have been just one of the pack if I had stayed with my siblings, but in all honesty, I am a princess in my present surroundings and being considered royalty is nothing to bark at.

I bring this up because I hear humans always discussing the joys of family and its benefits, and I listen to my mother and I get confused. Like for instance, what are in laws? We always have the TV on and sometimes I watch Westerns and hear about outlaws. I don't think they're the same as in laws although they don't seem very warm and friendly, either.

Another confusing thing is that two legged family members talk about taking care of one another when someone gets sick or very old, but when these same two legged family members talk about us, they say that when we get old or sick they will put us out of our misery. Woof! I don't like how that sounds. Who's miserable? We may have 4 legs but we can stand pain, too.

My mother shakes her head and says that blood is thicker than water. It sure looks that way and I'm a carnivore, so there's no argument from me, but she doesn't have her happy face on when she says that. I think it has something to do with blood, like in family relatives. I don't ever see the relatives because I'm not invited to visit. Has something to do with cats and the way I growl at other 4 legged creatures. I'm disinvited, although my bark is definitely worse than my bite. In fact, I don't have a bite, but when you weigh 6 lbs you have to make your presence known.

I love my family - my mother - and I have no complaints. Well, maybe one. It seems like there's always something more important on TV that she has to watch for a few brief minutes, when I give her my look of love stare that says I'm ready for a treat. Other than that, I think I've trained her pretty well and as far as families go, as I said, no complaints. Doggone unusual, huh?

55. ELEPHANTS: AGING WITH GRACE

Yes, elephants carry their trunks with them, but they never carry extra baggage. They never forget, but they always forgive, and that makes them far superior to us poor homo sapiens. They have strong family bonds, caring for all members as their own, in time of need, and that also gives them a leg or trunk up, wouldn't you say?

Of course I love Daisy, my little 6 lb Yorkie, but I have a small apartment and though the powers that be, claim to be pet friendly, there is a 20 lb weight limit, so you see my dilemma. I will have to love elephants from afar, and endeavor to understand and at times try hard to tolerate the humans who surround me.

The issue that I so often come up against is that of the pursed lip, otherwise known as the look of mean. Do you know what I mean? No pun intended. Maybe you've been more fortunate than I, and have managed to avoid both that facial expression and accompanying words, but I have not, and you remember that old adage about sticks and stones? Well I must admit that sometimes words cause a lot of pain and you wonder why they have been said. Words unsaid can also be painful and I will illustrate what I mean.

    For example, a neighbor has not spoken to me for 2 years because of some incident that I don't think occurred outside of her imagination and despite my efforts to apologize - in spite of this fact - I have been unsuccessful, and she still passes me in the hallway as if I were wearing my cloak of invisibility. Another neighbor, having damaged my car and not wanting to report it to the insurance company, and I foolishly agreeing to less money than from a subsequent actual estimate, is angry because I accepted less than the actual estimate, but wanted more than my original offer, and is not happy with me. Do I owe her an apology? Maybe, but first I have to flog myself for allowing her not to report the damage to my car.

    As I mentioned earlier, my complex is supposedly pet friendly but there are many less pets than people, and so we who hold the leashes bend over backwards to not stir up the ire of those who do not. So the other night I entered the elevator with Daisy at my side- she's not permitted to walk on the carpets but the elevator is not carpeted. However, when two women entered, I asked if they would prefer that I put Daisy in her carriage. They said they would and I did. As I was exiting the elevator, one woman said to the other, "I don't mind the dogs; It's the owners I don't like."

I am aging, but not dead or deaf and yes, I do bleed, and I thought of the pursed lips and the unkindness of these two women and I wonder, does being mean make someone feel better? I went to the zoo and spoke to the elephants and they said that if you want to feel good, you have to be good, and that's why they occasionally empty out their trunks and practice tusk love. Anyone know of an elephant friendly complex?

56. ONLY THE LONELY

Sometimes being alone is good. We all need time to think great thoughts, paint our toenails, ponder whether it's time for a brief cookie break, watch a TV show we won't admit we're addicted to, or shut our eyes for a quick forty winks. So, alone is more often than not, a good thing. Lonely - ah, that's something different altogether.

First of all, to make the difference between words perfectly clear, when we speak of being alone. what we mean is a choice we make for ourselves. For a variety of reasons, some of us need more alone time than do others. Some of us have more inner resources or prefer activities that are best accomplished on our own. It may simply be that we find our own company acceptable, and at times, preferable. This is not a matter of one option being good and the other option not so good. This is a case of what makes us feel comfortable, remembering that being alone is what we have chosen.

Lonely implies that we are alone and not by choice, but because we are in some way missing the company of others. There are many reasons for not having other people in our lives. Perhaps we would like to have many friends, but we know very few people, and making friends has always been difficult for us. On the other hand, maybe we expect too much of people, wanting them to meet our exacting standards. Perhaps we wear an aura of negativity and we're not much fun to be around. Or perhaps we have outlived many of our former friends, and friendships are not as easily formed as we age. A study designed to measure life satisfaction as we grow older, discovered that having a strong friend and or family support system, contributed more to life satisfaction, than any other factor.

Examining our faces, it is clear that lines are inevitable, so why not have lines that come from smiling? Remember those words from that famous commercial, "reach out and touch someone." A warm smile, heartfelt and contagious, can break the barriers that sometimes keep us apart. And don't worry if you don't get a smile in return. We're not going to allow any curmudgeons to keep us from growing older disgracefully. We are who we are, and as long as we don't try to change anyone else, we can be lonely grouches, or grouches surrounded by lots of other grouches like ourselves, who don't want to be alone.

57. MY CAR COMES CLEAN

The weather outside's delightful, but my windshield and all my windows are quite unsightful, so after many more months than we care to count, off we go to the car wash, a chore that for some reason, I always postpone. Actually, I have figured it out. It's car related and that means there will be - not so much a lot of problems - but rather lots of little annoyances I won't be able to solve. For starters, the intake person comes running out to the car to tell me that my antenna refuses to be detached from the car, and they can't take responsibility if the antenna bends or breaks. I suggest that they should bend, rather then break, the antenna. She gives me the look of love and off she goes, mumbling something about responsibility and I just laugh. No one takes responsibility for anything anymore. So tell me something I don't know.

Inauspicious start, but I need window wash fluid for my window washer and so I buy a bottle, which I am told has to be diluted, but Bill, the manager will do the filling up, if I ask. I ask and he takes the bottle from me, attempts to pour some into the fluid container, which is already full, I am informed. He steps into the car and the washers work for him like a charm.

I know my car does not love me but really, does it have to go out of its way to embarrass me? Anyway, when the hood is up, I notice lots of leaves and try to remove them, but Bill says he will send the car back to be re vacuumed. At last the car is returned, clean and shiny and Bill smiles a warm goodbye. Hasn't he observed that I am one of the growing older disgracefully crowd and he is therefore supposed to shake his head and smile superciliously at me?

I'm not paid to advertise, but I have to say that this car wash is off 590 and 19 in Clearwater and has definitely impacted on my fear of coming clean with my car. Now, if I could find a gas station whose employees don't think I'm feeble minded when I forget to screw my gas cap in place? Or even better, offer what used to be known as full service, so the screwing back is their responsibility. Oops. that word again. Let's go back to clean.

58. WHERE DID MY LITTLE WHEELS GO?

The time comes to all of us when we have to lose what is more than our transport. On the surface, it seems just a car but we know it's so much more than that. Suddenly, there goes our power to decide. Maybe we never went many places, but we went when we wanted, where we wanted and our decision was unilateral and man, didn't that feel good! Sometimes we had to wait for a cash infusion to gas up a little, but that was ok. Our car, our gas, our decision. Yummy!

We, who are growing older disgracefully, understand that being behind the wheel of what can be a deadly weapon, may affect more than ourselves, and unlike those who text and talk while in motion, our ability to multitask may be somewhat impaired.

Although if truth be told, I have some serious doubts about multitasking in general, and I'm not entirely convinced that age is always the culprit in vehicular loss of control. Have to do a little statistical googling to make that a definitive statement. In the meanwhile, I would accept that uncorrectable loss of vision and any impaction on my ability to see other cars, pedestrians or deer, or other animals crossing the road, would mean surrender of my handicapped parking, or any other parking space, forever.

So there go my spurts of impulse buying, although I think those faded away a long time ago. For financial reasons, shopping is no longer a pastime. I go to the grocery, not to save myself from starvation, but to add the little treats to which my little four legged friend and I have become accustomed. Not the same treats, of course, but the same principle. We are deserving and who is to say nay?

Actually, I will be more able to fund means of transport - senior buses, even taxicabs - -because I no longer pay car insurance, gas fill ups and car payments. I will be positively rich. Still, I will wake up some morning feeling positively bereft. I have just read of some health guru who will be lecturing in Sarasota tomorrow, and who promises inner peace, which will last probably longer than I will.

Too late to make arrangements. My car has been sent to the happy hunting grounds. I really need that blasted inner peace right now. Darn stupid for that guru to live in Sarasota. Lots more people need inner peace in Clearwater. I'm not sorry about the loss of my car. Sorry about the thoughtlessness of people. Maybe I could do a bicycle. Do they still sell training wheels? Wheels. Need wheels

59. RECIPE FOR LIVING

If you must have a recipe for just about everything that you do, obviously out of the box is not your style of life, and that's ok, so long as you're cognizant of just who you are. For instance, we were talking recipes one day and someone said she can't boil water without a recipe. That was a joke, I hope, because I'm one of those who believe that recipes are great if you're entering a contest, but I'm more one of those who- whatever is on hand goes into the pot-types. The most famous sushi chef in the world - and it doesn't matter if you don't like Sushi - is at the top of his class and he says that there are two things that are absolutely necessary if you hope to be a great chef. You must have a good nose and an equally good sense of taste.

I love what he says because smell and taste are vitally important in everything that we do, and without one or both, we find ourselves limited, and I am not just referring to the kitchen. Recipes, maps, a GPS and Robert's (or anybody else's) rules of order are anathema to some of us and make us feel constricted and wanting to break out of wherever we are. A popular song from my youth was built on lyrics saying, "Don't Fence Me In", and I loved that thought. Me and lots of other people who bought the albums.

Of course, someone has to make the rules, but who is that someone? Without any rules at all we would have anarchy, but without the ability to create or to think outside of the box, we would still be using legal sized yellow ruled pads and writing with lead pencils.

There has to be someone who tells us that what we want to do is impossible, that it has never been done before and that it just cannot be done. For some people, the words "it cannot be done" are akin to the actions of the picador who tosses a red cape across the bulls' face. These are the people who create their own recipes, be it in the kitchen or a garage or the top of a mountain.

Do you have a recipe for life or is just living your way, your secret recipe? Tell, tell, tell or maybe just show.

Evelyn Marder Levin

60. I S THICKER THAN

Once upon a time I had a sister - an older sister by 4 years - and we were close as 2 peas in a pod, except for the times when we weren't. Well, you might know how that goes. A little sibling rivalry, a little envy, a little adoration, mostly on my part, as her status changed in my eyes from icon to witch. But mostly she was the cat's meow and I wanted to look like her, dress like her, in fact if I could have been her that would have been perfect.

At a time when it was the fashion, she had curly hair and mine was straight. I was chubby but she started out nice and thin. However I got taller and thinner with long straight blond hair, and although I still idolized her, I was no longer the ugly duckling, except inside my brain. Our interests were very different. I was musical and she was into business and fashion and in my eyes, became an amazing success.

She married first. I wasn't enamored of her husband but apparently, neither was she, because they divorced about 10 years later. By then I had married and she had 2 sons and I had 3. Back to the peas in the pod. We remained close during all this time. Because of our friendship, we all spent much time together and I thought we always would. My sister remarried and we began to drift apart.

She was still my hero and having to emulate her as always, I divorced and remarried as had she. Only difference was that she married a wealthy, successful man and I married a con man. Our needs had changed and we saw one another infrequently. Before her remarriage, our roles had somewhat interchanged. She went through a bad patch and I had temporarily become the older sister.

I believe our final separation was the result of a substantial loan that she made to my husband, which he never paid back. I can understand her feelings and yet I cannot, since the unpaid loan has not impacted her life and I cannot cover it. My husband has destroyed my credit, still owes money to the immediate world, and has made me the recipient of his outstanding collection calls.

So now we are 2 old biddies who barely keep in contact with each other, except for birthdays and other possible state occasions. We have not seen one another in over a decade and even on the rare occasions when my sister travels with her son, to my part of the world, we do not meet because of age and travel logistics. So it would seem.

I could use a sister in my life - I have no daughters nor does she - and I miss the wonderful years of kinship we had. I will probably never see her again since that's still an up in the air question. If she is seeking retribution, she has it. I am the elderly poor we always read about and she is not.

So when we hang up the phone, I pick up a book or turn on the TV or go to my blog. As the song goes, "Regrets, I have a few," but my own song says, "It hasn't been all bad. Has it?" No, it hasn't. I've been lucky. I've had a 4 legged companion for the past 13 years, who shares my life, and I pray that we will take our last breaths together. Same prayer. Different cast of characters.

61. WHAT PRICE DIGNITY? RESPECT?

There's a question I've been asking myself recently. Actually, I ask myself lots of questions, but this one in particular, has been nagging at my brain with some frequency. Do we worry too much about our dignity? What is dignity, after all? It's a very subjective word and maybe it's overrated, in so far as what it means to us. Dignity could be defined in terms of the respect others show to us, as well as to the ways in which we respect ourselves. Respect. Another tricky word.

Actually, if we're among those persons who are growing older disgracefully, we shouldn't give a flying fig about what others think of us, and most especially those persons on whom we sometimes depend, like for instance, our offspring. I know, we gave them our help without being asked, but that more or less comes with the territory of parenting, good parenting, at least. "We didn't ask to be born". How often have we heard that plaintive refrain? And they're right, but we didn't ask to get old -it just comes with the territory- and I guess, maybe misguidedly at times, we thought that having cast our bread upon the waters, somehow that bread would come back to us.

Trust me, we know that asking for help is the pits, and makes us feel useless and undignified. Things we have been doing for years without any special thought, become a step by step process. We used to jump out of a car, and now we have to lift one foot at a time to conquer a door sill. This same car that was our lifeline has become our nemesis. The road signs have diminished, along with our vision, and everyone on the road is in a race against time. Or so it seems.

In a society where technology rules, our years of experience and acquired wisdom seems without value, but who sets the standards of value? We have as much right as anyone to set the standards, and that's where self-respect plays a vital role. The habits of a lifetime, habits of decency and empathy and concern for our fellow men and women are etched on our being, and not subject to electronic deletion. So there!

62. HAPPINESS

Is not a given. It's out there someplace, and you may have to struggle to find it, but once you learn the way, you may get side tracked from time to time, only you will never lose one another again.

Sounds easy? Well, of course it's not. Easy peasy is only for TV commercials. The real world is a little more complex. First of all, happiness is not a universal. One size definitely does not fit all. For me and lots of us who are growing older disgracefully, when we offer felicitations for the new year, we do not say, Happy New Year, we say Healthy New Year, because that is at the top of our agenda. Can't have the first without the second - no way, Jose - and we have learned through life experience.

Is that true for everyone? Don't know. Can't say.

I have only lived the life I'm living and when I was younger, when my body bent to the wishes of my mind, when pain was a distant or rare stranger, when I made plans before I got out of bed in the morning and followed through without a second thought - Well, to be honest, I probably thought that happiness was a trip to the moon in a balloon or some other excursion to fantasy land, because I owned the world or at least the parts of the world that I inhabited. I was the captain of my soul, my body and anything else I could lay claim to. Mary Poppins, Harry Potter, even Superman, were all part of my life and the strong physical foundation that supported me. There was an occasional crack - nothing serious - but I was unlike any other, I was strong.

I was young and I didn't have to delve within myself to keep occasional thoughts of doubt at bay. Mind control? Really! Next you'll talk of crystal balls and spirits. My definitions were changing. Finding shoes to match my handbag? No, the ability to get in my car and drive to where I want, when I want, and not have to adjust my schedule to the community bus. That was happiness, predicated on my state of health, so I could maintain my independence and do as I pleased.

From this small example I was able to expand my horizons. My environment was nice, exceptionally so, and I had enough room to share my living space with my long, long time pet and my exercise equipment (which I use) and my computer and my TV and my favorite rocking chair in which I read. I could write, read, chat with my neighbors when so inclined and I had a focus in my life.

I pray for a quality of life rather than great quantity. I want to be able to continue with my - at times - convoluted roll out of bed, to find the humor in most issues of life, to tell my four legged girlfriend how much I love her, and I guess I will have found happiness. No, no - I don't guess. I know. I have found happiness. Like my keys, it disappears from time to time, but when I get to the door, both appear and we're no longer apart.

I hope you find your happiness. I hope, I hope, I hope.

Made in the USA
Charleston, SC
30 April 2015